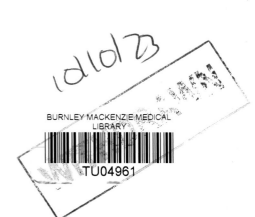

Alberto Rosenblatt
Renaud Bollens
Baldo Espinoza Cohen

Manual of Laparoscopic Urology

Foreword by Claude Schulman

With 334 Figures

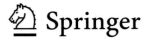 Springer

ISBN 978-3-540-74726-0
e-ISBN 978-3-540-74727-7

Library of Congress Control Number:
2007935176

Alberto Rosenblatt
Albert Einstein Jewish Hospital (HIAE)
Av. Albert Einstein, 627/701
São Paulo 05651-901
Brazil
albrose1@gmail.com

Renaud Bollens
Erasme Hospital
University Clinics of Brussels
Route de Lennik 808 B
1070 Brussels
Belgium
renaud.bollens@ulb.ac.be

Baldo Espinoza Cohen
Hospital Clinico Regional de Antofagasta
Hospital Militar del Norte
General Borgoño 957
Antofagasta
Chile
baldo_doc@yahoo.es

Cover design: Frido Steinen-Broo, EStudio Calamar, Spain

Printed on acid-free paper
9 8 7 6 5 4 3 2 1

springer.com

Effort only fully releases its reward
after a person refuses to quit.

Napoleon Hill

Foreword

Fellows from all over the world come to the Department of Urology at the University Clinics of Brussels at Erasme Hospital to learn or improve their skills in laparoscopy, a very rapidly expanding new surgical approach for most urological procedures traditionally performed by open surgery.

The urologists, whether experienced or in training, come to familiarise themselves with the different laparoscopic procedures, but it can take quite a long time to see all of the various procedures, and it can be especially difficult to learn the numerous tips and tricks that are used by expert laparoscopists.

The idea of writing a manual of laparoscopic urology grew progressively during the fellowship of Dr. Alberto Rosenblatt and Dr. Baldo Espinoza in our department in 2006. Their main objective was to compile valuable and difficult to find information and offer this instructive and well-illustrated material to the urologic community.

This manual was conceived in a very practical way and highlights the step-by-step approach used in each procedure. The text also calls attention to the "little details" that make all the difference when it comes to putting the steps into practice.

Of course, every expert in laparoscopy or open surgery has his own technique and his particular variety of practical advice. The techniques that are illustrated in this book are the standard ones used by Dr. Renaud Bollens at Erasme Hospital and by the different members of the department's team under his expertise.

Essentially, this comprehensive Manual of Laparoscopic Urology is an expansion of personal notes that should be extremely helpful to all of those interested in learning this challenging surgical technique.

December 2007
Brussels, Belgium

Professor Claude Schulman

Preface

The excitement of moving into the field of laparoscopic surgery can be quickly overshadowed by the realization of how long it takes to acquire the skills needed to master the technique. Indeed, laparoscopic surgery requires a very good knowledge of anatomy as well as fairly good manual dexterity. Skills can be developed by practicing basic laparoscopic sutures in the "black box" or by training in a virtual environment, but it is only by performing real laparoscopic operations that a surgeon can become truly competent.

However, learning time can be reduced by gaining an understanding of the small details and "tricks of the trade" that laparoscopic experts utilize and that increasingly facilitate the laparoscopic procedure.

The aim of this manual of urologic laparoscopy is to provide urologists and surgeons who are willing to master the techniques with a time-tested and reliable source of practical information on laparoscopic surgery.

Although the focus of this manual is on urological procedures, plenty of valuable technical information that can be applied to any laparoscopic specialty has been included.

Like a mentor, this manual will guide the laparoscopic surgeon through every aspect of the laparoscopic procedure, from the equipment's settings to the correct positioning of the needle on the needle holder. Every urologic procedure is described in a step-by-step sequence of events, and the text is supplemented with innumerous tips, colored illustrations, and high-definition pictures depicting the main steps.

By following this well-illustrated sequence of surgical steps, readers can be confident in their ability to master the laparoscopic technique.

August 2007   *Alberto Rosenblatt, M.D.*
São Paulo, Brazil

Contents

Section I

General Laparoscopic Information

Chapter 1

Fundamentals of Laparoscopic Surgery

Contents

Introduction

The use of laparoscopic surgery has rapidly expanded since the laparoscope merged with the video camera in the mid-1980s. Since then, significant developments of laparoscopic equipment and instruments have been made. Along with the technology, surgical skills have also improved with the incorporation of advanced laparoscopic techniques, allowing surgeons to safely perform a multitude of laparoscopic interventions. Apart from the state-of-the-art equipment and surgical expertise, laparoscopic procedures are usually technically demanding, requiring well-trained operative teams and good coordination with an anesthesiologist well versed in laparoscopy. Putting everything to work in perfect combination can make the difference between a safe, efficient operation and a long, difficult procedure that will increase the risk of perioperative and postoperative complications.

General Considerations

Physiologic Effects of Pneumoperitoneum

Carbon dioxide (CO_2) is the gas commonly used for inflating the abdomen. Once inside the abdominal space, it is rapidly absorbed across the peritoneal membrane into the circulatory system. In the blood, carbonic acid is produced leading to respiratory acidosis, but this condition is attenuated due to the absorption of the CO_2 by body buffers. However, during long laparoscopic procedures, body buffers become saturated and hypercapnia or respiratory acidosis develops. At this point, the lungs become responsible for the absorption and release of CO_2 from the body buffers. Although this condition can be corrected by the anesthesiologist, the associated effects of pneumoperitoneum pressure on the different organ systems can potentiate significant clinical disturbances (see Pneumoperitoneum and Potential Clinical Outcomes).

The pressure effects of pneumoperitoneum:

- Increases intra-abdominal pressure
- Decreases cardiac output and stroke volume
- Decreases femoral venous blood flow and venous return
- Reduces renal perfusion and intraoperative urine output
- Decreases respiratory compliance and increases airway pressure
- Increases intracranial pressure

Pneumoperitoneum and Potential Clinical Outcomes

Pulmonary System

- High peak airway pressures leading to an increased risk of barotrauma and/or pneumothorax
- Superior displacement of the diaphragm leading to an increase in Pco_2 and/or a decrease in Po_2 levels
- Decreased pulmonary compliance and vital capacity leading to an increase in Pco_2 and/or a decrease in Po_2 levels

Circulatory System

- Increased central venous pressure, systemic vascular resistance, capillary wedge pressure, and mean arterial pressure leading to an increase in cardiac work
- Indirect effects on the sympathetic system, renin–angiotensin system, and vasopressin leading to an increase in blood pressure and cardiac output
- Indirect effects of hypercapnia, such as arteriolar dilation and myocardial depression leading to a decrease in blood pressure
- Vasovagal response caused by a rapid stretch of the peritoneum leading to bradycardia and occasionally a decrease in blood pressure

- Coagulation disturbances, such as lower extremity venous stasis leading to deep venous thrombosis (DVT) and pulmonary embolism (PE)

Renal System

- Reduced renal blood flow and glomerular filtration rate leading to a diminished urine output (direct pressure on kidney and renal vein)
- Increased release of renin with sodium retention
- Release of antidiuretic hormone (ADH), increasing water reabsorption in the distal tubules

Gastrointestinal System

- Decreased sympathetic response leading to less ileus paralyticus

Central Nervous System

- Increased intracranial pressure leading to reduced central perfusion pressure

Immunologic System

- Less pronounced immune suppression
- Fast return of cytokine levels to normal values

General Advantages of Laparoscopy

- Small incision
- Minimal pain
- Attenuated stress response
- Earlier return to ambulation
- Reduced hospital stay
- Fast recovery

Laparoscopic Contraindications

Intraperitoneal Access

Absolute Contraindications

- Acute peritonitis
- Severe chronic pulmonary obstructive disease
- Congestive heart failure
- Abdominal wall infections
- Bleeding diatheses
- Intestinal obstruction
- Malignant ascites
- Acute glaucoma
- Increased cranial pressure
- Ventriculoperitoneal and peritoneojugular shunts (increased CO_2 absorption and acidosis)

Relative Contraindications

- Severe chronic pulmonary obstructive disease
- Extensive prior abdominal surgery
- Aneurysms of the aorta or iliac arteries
- Intestinal obstruction
- Pelvic fibrosis (previous radiation therapy and previous hip replacement surgery due to sealant leakage)
- Organomegaly
- Severe diaphragmatic hernia (risk of CO_2 leakage into the mediastinum)
- Pregnancy

Extraperitoneal Access

Relative Contraindications

- Prior lower abdominal surgery
- Prior pelvic surgery
- Prior inguinal hernia surgical repair

General Complications of Laparoscopy

Injury to Adjacent Organs

- Bowel puncture (see Veress Needle Introduction)
- Bowel wall thermal injury
- Bleeding from solid organs (liver and spleen)
- Bladder perforation
- Uterus puncture

Vascular Injuries

- Abdominal wall vessels

> **TIP**
>
> *An injury to the abdominal wall vessels is usually visible as blood dripping from one of the trocars and/or blood seen on the surface of abdominal structures. The usual cause of the bleeding is an iatrogenic injury to the inferior epigastric artery or one of its branches. The bleeding can be controlled with the application of direct pressure using the involved trocar, coagulation of the vessel with the bipolar grasper, or a laparoscopic-guided or open suture ligation tied over a gauze bolster to tamponade the bleeding site.*

- Intra-abdominal large and small vessels

> **TIP**
>
> *The right common iliac artery lies directly below the umbilicus. (see Veress Needle Introduction)*

Access Complications

- Port site hernia
- Wound infection

- Port site seeding of tumor cells

Pneumoperitoneum Complications

- Pneumothorax
- Pneumomediastinum
- Subcutaneous emphysema
- Gas embolus

Special Considerations

Anesthesia Problems in Laparoscopic Surgery

Trendelenburg Position

- Increases intracranial and intraocular pressures, which may lead to cerebral edema, retinal detachment, and even blindness (especially the long-lasting extreme head-down position for pelvic and lower abdominal procedures)
- Increases intrathoracic pressure, central venous pressure, capillary wedge pressure, and mean arterial pressure leading to an increase in cardiac work
- Increases venous return, which in combination with pneumoperitoneum may lead to congestive heart failure and even acute myocardial infarction

Hypercapnia

When hypercapnia occurs:
- Reduce the intra-abdominal pressure or stop the procedure until Pco_2 decreases
- Decrease the angle of the Trendelenburg position
- Increase the minute volume of ventilation

> **TIP**
>
> *To avoid the risk of subcutaneous emphysema and hypercapnia, never suture the skin around the trocar when fixing it.*

CO₂ Embolism

Usually occurs due to misplacement of the Veress needle:
- Into a vessel
- Into a parenchymal organ (mainly the liver)
- Hypovolemia is a risk factor

Signs of CO₂ Embolism

- Profound hypotension
- Cyanosis
- Arrhythmias
- Asystole
- Immediate increase of end-tidal CO_2 accompanied by a sudden decline in oxygen saturation and then a marked decrease in end-tidal CO_2 due to cardiovascular collapse

When a CO_2 embolism is suspected, the following measures must be taken immediately:
- Stop insufflation and deflate the pneumoperitoneum
- Place the patient in a left lateral head-down position (this will enable the gas embolus to move into the right ventricular apex, preventing its entry into the pulmonary artery)
- Increase minute ventilation and 100% in-tidal O_2 administration
- Introduce a central venous catheter to enable aspiration of the gas
- Administer cardiopulmonary resuscitation in case of asystole
- Administer hyperbaric oxygen therapy, if available

TIP

Most cases of suspected gas embolism will resolve with the first two measures above.

Recovery Period

Extended postoperative mechanical ventilation may sometimes be needed until all extra CO_2 has been eliminated:

- Following prolonged laparoscopic procedures
- When high intra-abdominal insufflation pressure is applied
- When extensive subcutaneous emphysema is present

Urine output must be carefully controlled:

- Following prolonged laparoscopic procedures
- When high intra-abdominal insufflation pressure is applied

Postoperative Nausea and Vomiting

Etiology

- Mechanical pressure to gut and stomach
- Stretching of vagal nerve endings in the peritoneum
- Vasodilatation of the cerebral vessels by CO_2, consequently raising the intracranial pressure

Prophylaxis

- Antiemetics
- Ondansetron, 4 mg administered intravenously just before the end of surgery
- Dexamethasone in combination with Ondansetron to extend the duration of antiemesis

Pain Management

- Evacuation of residual gas before trocar removal
- Opioid analgesia
- Local anesthetic infiltration of port sites
- Preemptive analgesia

Technical Considerations

Preinsufflation Checklist

- CO_2 tank is full or an extra tank is available
- Gas valve on the cylinder is open
- Laparoscopic tower is switched on and equipment is operational
- Insufflator is operational and settings are correct (see Insufflator Checklist)
- In-line filter is connected between insufflator and insufflation tubing
- Electrosurgical unit is operational and settings are correct
- Instruments are compatible with electrocautery and adequately insulated
- Bipolar and monopolar scissor pedals are connected and operational
- Laparoscope image is white balanced
- Suction device is operational (suction and irrigation tubing are connected and working)
- Veress needle tip retracts properly

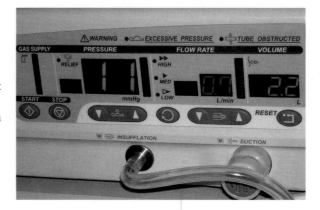

FIG. 1
Insufflator settings

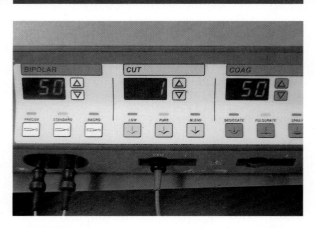

FIG. 2
Electrosurgical unit

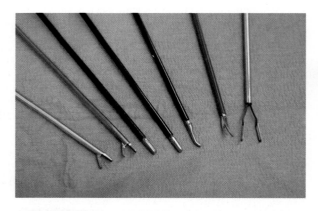

FIG. 3
Instruments for laparoscopic surgery

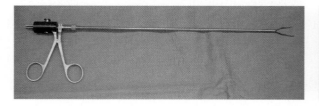

FIG. 4
Bipolar grasper

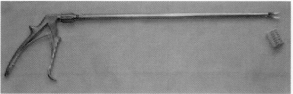

FIG. 5
Ethicon™ clip applier (10 mm) and clips

- An extra pair of scissors is available

Insufflator Checklist

- Maximum pressure on the insufflator is set to 12 mmHg
- Pressure is set according to the following:
  - Initiate with high pressure when performing an extraperitoneal laparoscopic radical prostatectomy or when using the open access technique
  - Initiate with low pressure when using the Veress needle (closed access) technique
- CO_2 flow rate is set to 35 L/min (Fig. 1)
- Safety valve pressure is set to 35 mmHg

Insufflator Tips

- Intra-abdominal pressure for safe trocar introduction should be equal to or higher than 10 mmHg.

> **TIP**
>
> *Pressure is the most important parameter.*

- Intra-abdominal volume for safe trocar introduction should be equal to or higher than 2.5 L.

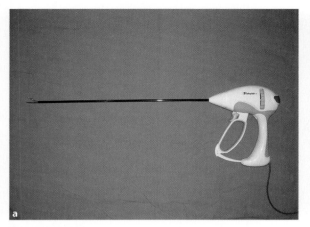

FIG. 6

a LigaSure™ 5 mm (Tyco Healthcare). **b** LigaSure at bladder pedicle

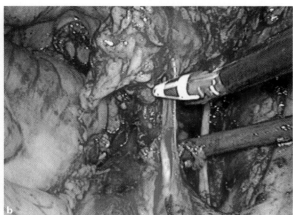

Electrosurgical Unit Settings

- Monopolar Coagulation set to 50 Watts (Fig. 2)
- Cutting set to 0
- Bipolar Coagulation set to 50 Watts
- Auto stop set to Off

Instruments for Laparoscopic Surgery

Basic Instruments (see Fig. 3)

- Needle holder
- Bipolar grasper (Fig. 4)
- Monopolar scissors

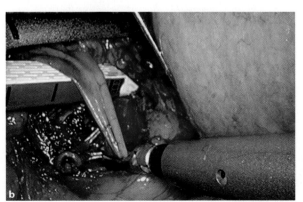

FIG. 7

a Multifire Endo GIA™ 30 12-mm stapler. **b** Endo GIA stapling renal vein

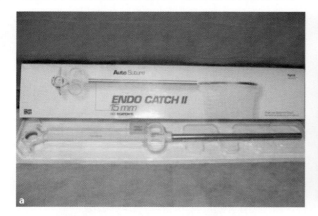

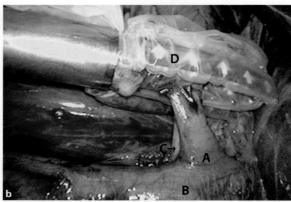

FIG. 8

a Endo Catch II 15 mm (Autosuture). **b** Renal vein (A); V. cava (B); Right renal artery (C); Kidney inside Endobag (D)

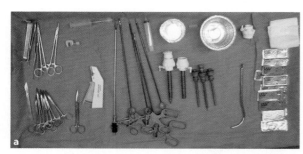

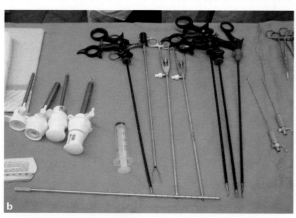

FIG. 9

a Laparoscopic instruments/trocars for radical prostatectomy. **b** Laparoscopic instruments/trocars for promontory fixation

- Graspers

Other Instruments for Vessel and Tissue Ligation

- Clip applier forceps (non-disposable) (Fig. 5)
- Laparoscopic sealer/divider instrument

TIP

The LigaSure™ 5 mm (Tyco Healthcare) has a small tip suitable for tissue dissection, and the sealing and dividing function is hand-controlled. (Fig. 6a,b)

- Endo GIA™ 30 12-mm stapler (Autosuture) (Fig. 7a,b)

Specimen Retrieval Device

- Endobag (Fig. 8a,b)

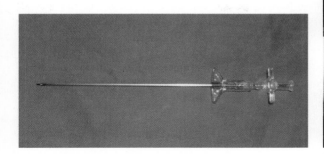

FIG. 10
Disposable Veress needle

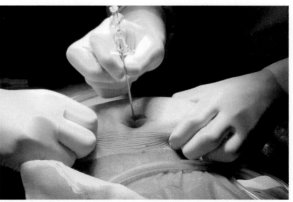

FIG. 11
Veress needle introduction

Laparoscopic Instruments Table (see Fig. 9a,b)

Veress Needle Introduction (Closed Access)

The Veress needle can be disposable or reusable (Fig. 10).
The blunt tip of the needle retracts when it is pressed against a tough structure, exposing its sharp edge. After the needle passes through the abdominal wall layers, the blunt tip is deployed, preventing damage to the abdominal structures. The CO_2 gas for the abdominal insufflation passes through the hollow cannula of the Veress needle.

> **TIP**
>
> *The maximum flow through the needle is 0.2 L/min due to its internal diameter.*

While introducing the needle, it is important to feel it passing through the layers of the abdominal wall. The initial thrust is at the level of the external oblique/rectus fascia, followed by the transversalis fascia and peritoneum.

> **TIP**
>
> *As the needle enters the peritoneal cavity, a click sound can often be heard, meaning the blunt tip has sprung forward.*

It is preferable to avoid introduction of the Veress needle in the vicinity of a previous abdominal scar.

> **TIP**
>
> *When bowel adhesions are suspected, the Veress needle is not used, and the fascia is opened under direct vision (i.e., open access); the peritoneum should be digitally entered and the adhesions carefully released with gentle digital movements.*

Introduction Technique for Pelvic Laparoscopic Procedures

A subumbilical incision is made 50% larger than the diameter of the trocar that will be inserted. The abdominal wall is elevated by manually grasping the skin and subcutaneous tissue (Fig. 11).

The Veress needle is grasped by the shaft like a dart and then passed into the incision perpendicularly to the abdominal wall. Following introduction, two tests are performed in sequence to confirm that the needle is inside the peritoneal cavity (Fig. 12).

1. Initially, a 20-mL syringe is connected to the needle, and the plunger is drawn out to test for the presence of air or blood. If blood is aspirated, a vessel was punctured and conversion to open surgery should be done without removal of the Veress needle. In the case that gas and/or a yellow or cloudy fluid are aspirated, the needle is placed inside the lumen of the bowel. The needle is then removed and replaced in the correct position. The optic is reintroduced, and the puncture of the bowel must be found and laparoscopically repaired. In this particular situation, a prosthesis should not be placed due to the risk of bacterial contamination.

2. Then, the syringe is filled with 20 mL of air. It is reconnected to the Veress needle, the air is injected, and the plunger is drawn out to test for the presence of air. *No air* should return to the syringe (if air returns, the needle is placed in a closed location and most probably in the preperitoneal space). The insufflation tubing is connected to the Veress needle, the stopcock is opened, and the abdomen is insufflated. Initiating with a low flow is recommended to avoid damage to a vital structure in case the needle is mispositioned. Switch to high flow if the intra-abdominal pressure is low and the insufflation pressure is increasing at a steady and normal level along with a tympanic percussion of the liver area. Then, the needle is removed and the primary trocar is introduced perpendicularly to the abdominal wall.

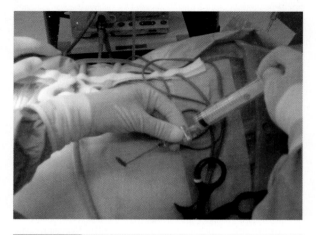

FIG. 12
Syringe is connected to Veress needle

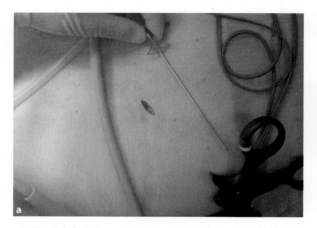

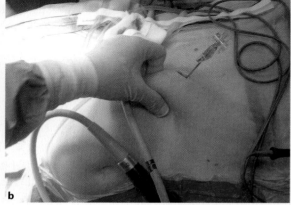

FIG. 13
a Subcostal incision. **b** Needle introduction through the incision

Technique of Laparoscopic Trocar Introduction

Types of Trocars

Trocars can be disposable or reusable and are available in different sizes (2 mm, 5 mm, 10 mm, 12 mm, and 15 mm). The obturator tip may be bladed or blunt, and the blunt tip may be associated with a lower incidence of injury to intraperitoneal structures and vessels of the abdominal wall (Fig. 14).

> **TIP**
>
> *Always check for a sharp tip on reusable trocars; unsharpened tips will result in a forceful thrust, increasing the risk of vessel or organ injury during laparoscopic access.*

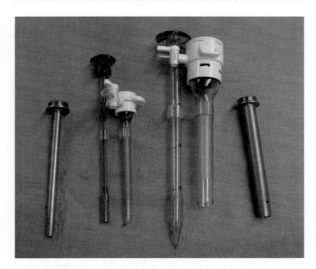

FIG. 14
Disposable blunt tip and reusable trocars

At the end of the laparoscopic procedure, the aponeurosis of trocar sites 10 mm or larger should be closed to avoid the occurrence of incisional hernias. The risk of hernias may be reduced by the utilization of the blunt tip trocar.

Trocar Positioning

The primary camera port preferably should be in line with the structure of interest (for example, the renal hilum during a laparoscopic nephrectomy), and at a 45° angle to the area of interest. The working ports (right and left hand) should be on either side of the camera port and at an adequate distance from each other and from the camera, preventing the crossing of the instruments. The smaller diameter trocar is usually positioned at the surgeon's dominant hand side, and the larger trocar is for the nondominant one. This is to prevent instrument shaking while performing sensitive tasks, which are usually exerted by the dominant hand. The secondary trocar placement site is marked by pressing a finger on the abdominal wall, and the indentation is internally viewed with the optic, allowing the insertion of all secondary trocars under direct laparoscopic visualization.

Introduction Technique for Upper Tract Laparoscopic Procedures

A cutaneous incision is made 50% larger than the diameter of the trocar that will be inserted. This is done two fingerbreadths below the costal margin arch, at the level of the lateral border of the rectus muscle. The abdominal wall is elevated by manually grasping the skin and subcutaneous tissue, and the Veress needle is introduced through the incision (Fig. 13a,b).

The Veress needle must be introduced perpendicularly to the plane of the patient

> **TIP**
>
> *For the right side, the needle can be introduced at an angle of 30° caudally to the abdominal wall to avoid liver puncture.*

After introduction, the procedures to confirm the correct placement of the needle are the same as for the pelvic laparoscopic surgery.

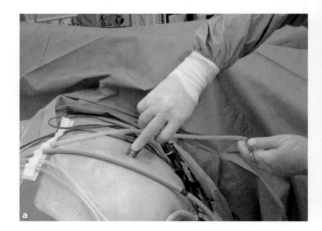

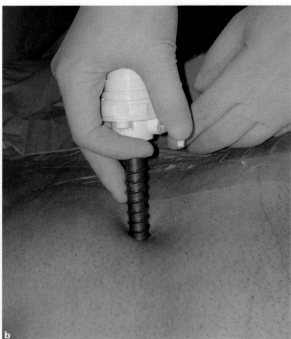

FIG. 15

a Trocar introduction (see middle finger position). **b** Trocar introduction

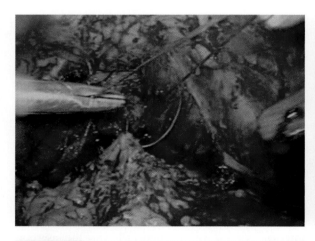

FIG. 16

The thread is straightened out

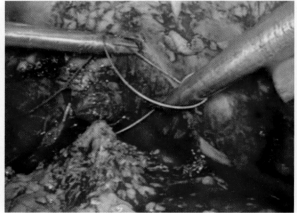

FIG. 17

Half loop open with both needle holders in close proximity

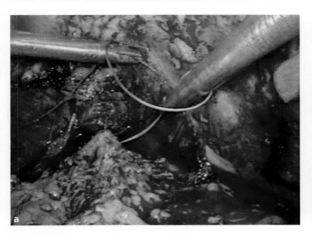
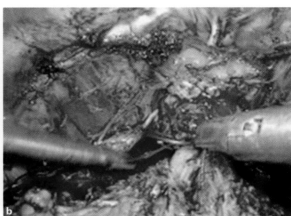

FIG. 18

a Left needle holder advances. **b** Right needle holder moves out of the loop

Trocar Introduction

Pneumoperitoneum should be adequate. The skin incision is made 50% larger than the diameter of the trocar. The trocar is firmly grasped against the palm of the hand to arm the device; the middle finger is extended for further insertion control, and the trocar is introduced with a firm and constant screwing motion (Fig. 15a,b).

The trocar should be inserted perpendicularly to the abdominal wall, and the insertion angle can be changed as soon as the tip pierces the peritoneum.

Following trocar placement and obturator removal, the trocar valve is briefly opened to check for egress of gas, confirming it is correctly placed inside the abdomen. The insufflator line is then connected to the trocar.

Laparoscopic Suturing Techniques

Basic Suturing

- The left needle holder grasps the thread.
- The thread is straightened out by pulling with the right needle holder.

- The axis of the thread is kept perpendicular to the left needle holder to facilitate loop construction (Fig. 16).
- A half loop is made.
- The left needle holder stays in close proximity to the right one to keep the loop opened (Fig. 17).
- The left needle holder advances forward, and the right needle holder moves out of the half loop (Fig. 18a,b).

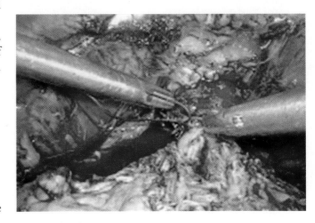

FIG. 19

Left needle holder grabs the open loop

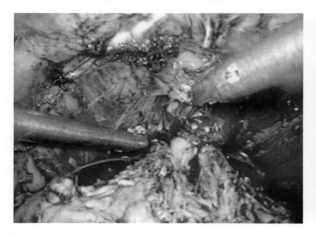

FIG. 20
The knot is closed

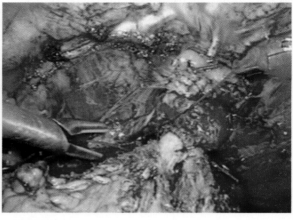

FIG. 21
Left needle holder swiftly grabs proximal thread

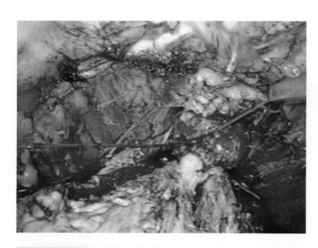

FIG. 22
Threads are pulled out, and the knot is tied

TIP

Do not pull with the right needle holder before the second knot is tied to avoid loosening the knot.

- The knot is completed by advancing the right needle holder forward, and the left needle holder pulls in toward the trocar.

TIP

To avoid intra-abdominal injures, never pull the thread by the needle.

Advanced Suturing

- When the first knot loosens, the left needle holder grabs the open loop, and the right needle holder grabs the distal thread (Fig. 19).
- The left needle holder gently pulls the loop to close the knot (Fig. 20).
- The left needle holder swiftly grabs the proximal thread while the right needle holder keeps the distal thread tensioned (Fig. 21).
- Both thread ends are pulled out to tie the knot (Fig. 22).

Suggested Readings

1. Sriprasad S, Yu DF: Positional anatomy of vessels that may be damaged at laparoscopy: new access criteria based on CT and ultrasonography to avoid vascular injury. J Endourol 2006 Jul; 20(7):498–503.

2. Hamade AM, Butt I: Closed blunt-trocar 5 mm-port for primary cannulation in laparoscopic surgery: a safe technique. Surg Laparosc Endosc Percutan Tech 2006 Jun; 16(3):156–160.

3. Jean JMCH de la Rosette, Inderbir SG: Laparoscopic Urologic Surgery in Malignancies. Springer, 2005.

4. Saber AA, Meslemani AM: Safety zones for anterior abdominal wall entry during laparoscopy: a CT scan mapping of epigastric vessels. Ann Surg 2004 Feb; 239(2):182–185.

5. Shalhav AL, Barret E: Transperitoneal laparoscopic renal surgery using blunt 12-mm trocar without fascial closure. J Endourol 2002 Feb; 16(1):43–46.

6. Rist M, Hemmerling TM: Influence of pneumoperitoneum and patient positioning on preload and splanchnic blood volume in laparoscopic surgery of the lower abdomen. J Clin Anesth 2001; 13:244–249.

7. Philips PA, Amaral JF: Abdominal access complications in laparoscopic surgery. J Am Coll Surg 2001; 19:525–536.

8. Odeberg-Wernerman S: Laparoscopic surgery – effects on circulatory and respiratory physiology: an overview. Eur J Surg Suppl 2000; 585:4–11.

9. Kashtan J, Green JF: Hemodynamic effects of increased abdominal pressure. J Surg Res 1981; 30:249–255.

10. Chapron CM, Pierre F: Major vascular injuries during gynecologic laparoscopy. J Am Coll Surg 1997; 185:461–465.

11. Riza ED, Deshmukh AS: An improved method of securing abdominal wall bleeders during laparoscopy. J Laparoendosc Surg 1995; 5:37–40.

12. Vasquez JM: Vascular complications of laparoscopic surgery. J Am Assoc Gynecol Laparosc 1994; 1:163–167.

13. Loris J: *Anesthetic Management of Laparoscopy*, 4th ed.. New York, Churchill Livingstone, 1994.

Section II

Laparoscopic Surgery for Malignant Urological Disorders

Chapter 2

Transperitoneal Laparoscopic Radical Nephrectomy

Contents

Introduction

Laparoscopic radical nephrectomy (LRN) is the surgical treatment of choice for patients presenting with early stage (T1) renal cell carcinoma. The laparoscopic approach has many advantages compared with open radical nephrectomy, including decreased blood loss, less pain, faster postoperative recovery, and improved cosmetics. Furthermore, this minimally invasive approach parallels the open technique in oncologic efficacy. The laparoscopic procedure has been increasingly used for higher stage tumors even though the use of the technique on large tumors has not yet been proved safe. Urologic surgeons with advanced laparoscopic skills are now able to manage highly selected patients with locally advanced disease and tumors with renal vein or vena cava thrombi. For selected kidney tumors less than 4 cm, current trends in organ preservation favor laparoscopic partial nephrectomy (see Chap. 3).

Preoperative Preparation

Before a patient consents to a laparoscopic nephrectomy, it is important to discuss the specific risks of the surgery, including the potential need to convert to the traditional open operation if difficulties arise.

The patient is admitted to the hospital the day before the surgery for bowel preparation, which includes 2 L of Colopeg® (1 envelope/L) p.o. and a Fleet® enema. Fasting starts at midnight before surgery. Thromboprophylaxis protocol is implemented with good hydration, placement of compressive elastic stockings on the lower extremities, and low-molecular-weight heparin. Enoxaparin (Clexane®, Lovenox®) 40 mg sc 1 × day or nadroparin (Flaxiparine®, Fraxiparin®) 0.6 mL sc 1 ×

day is initiated on day 1 after the surgery and continued daily until the patient is discharged from the hospital. In selected cases, the treatment is continued for 30 days after the procedure. Patients also receive antibiotic prophylaxis with a single preoperative dose of intravenous second-generation cephalosporin, unless they are allergic to penicillin. Blood type and crossmatch are determined.

Patient Positioning and Initial Preparation

The patient is initially positioned supine for intravenous access, induction of general anesthesia, and endotracheal intubation. An orogastric tube is placed and the stomach decompressed to avoid puncture during trocar placement and to allow additional space during abdominal insufflation. An 18Fr Foley catheter with 10 mL in the balloon is introduced for decompression of the bladder. During skin preparation, the entire flank and abdomen are included in case conversion to an open procedure is required. The umbilicus is placed over the break in the operating table, and the patient is positioned in a modified lateral decubitus position.

> **TIP**
>
> *For a left-side nephrectomy, the patient is placed in a strict lateral decubitus position.*

The table can be flexed as needed, or an inflatable balloon is positioned under the patient at the level of the umbilicus. Padding is used to support the buttocks and dorsum, and all potential pressure points are cushioned. An axillary roll is placed to prevent brachial plexus injury, and the arms should be positioned as far away from the trunk as possible so as not to disturb the movement of the operative team. The patient is held in position with strips of cloth tape (Fig. 1a,b).

The surgeon operates from the abdominal side of the patient, and the first assistant is placed caudally to the surgeon. The laparoscopic cart is positioned at the back of the patient's chest with the operative team facing the video monitor. The instruments table is positioned behind the operative team, and the assistant is positioned higher than the surgeon to prevent the laparoscopic instruments from conflicting (Fig. 2a–d).

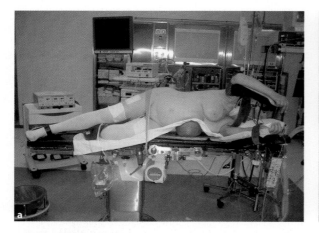 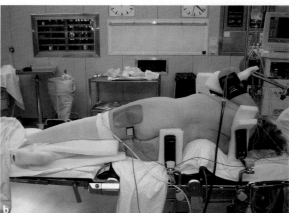

FIG. 1

a Patient position. **b** Padding

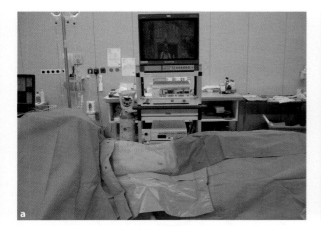

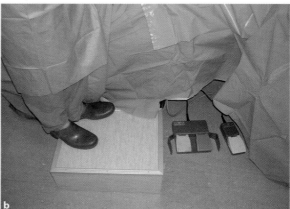

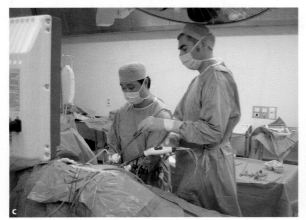

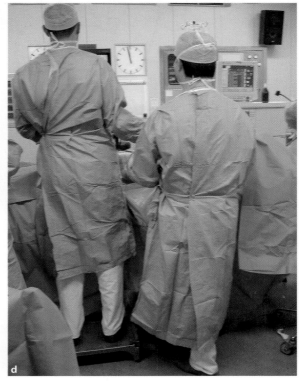

FIG. 2

a Patient and laparoscopic cart. **b** Steps below assistant.
c Instruments table behind operative team. **d** Operative
team's position

Trocars and Laparoscopic Instruments

Right-side nephrectomy:
- 2 × 11 mm (optic 0° and bipolar grasper)
- 3 × 5 mm (monopolar scissors, suction device, and liver retractor grasper)

Left-side nephrectomy:
- 2 × 11 mm (optic 0°, bipolar grasper, and 10-mm clip applier)
- 2 × 5 mm (scissors and suction device)
- Monopolar round-tipped scissors, bipolar grasper, liver retractor grasper, 5-mm suction device, 10-mm clip applier (non-disposable), needle drivers (2), and 10-mm laparoscopic optic 0°

Access and Port Placement

Four ports are generally enough to perform the procedure, although a fifth trocar may be necessary for liver retraction during a right-side nephrectomy (Fig. 3). Before trocars are placed, the abdomen is insufflated using a Veress needle.

TIP

In case of previous surgery, the Veress needle is not inserted, and the open access technique is used to place the first trocar.

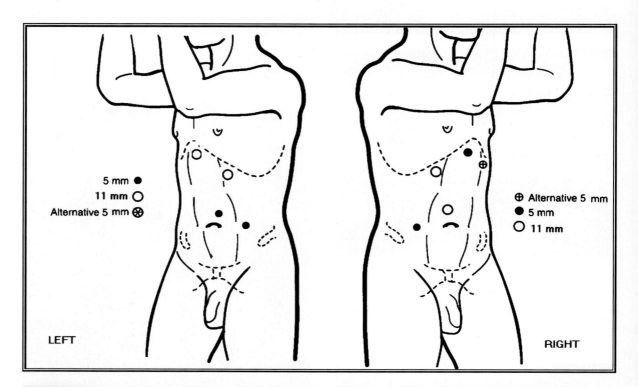

FIG. 3

Access and port placement (This figure was published in Wein: Campbell-Walsh Urology, 9th ed., Copyright Elsevier)

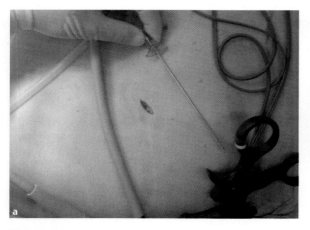

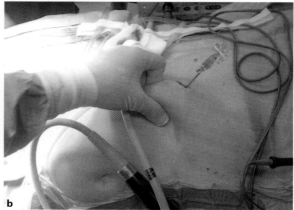

FIG. 4

a Cutaneous incision below costal margin. **b** Insertion of Veress needle

Veress Needle

A cutaneous incision is made two fingerbreadths below the costal margin arch, at the level of the lateral border of the rectus muscle (Fig. 4a,b).

> **TIP**
>
> *The skin incision should be 50% larger than the diameter of the 11-mm trocar.*

The Veress needle is introduced through the incision (see Chap. 1, Veress Needle Introduction).

First Port (11 mm, optic 0°)

Once pneumoperitoneum is established, the Veress needle is removed, and the 11-mm trocar is introduced through the same incision, perpendicularly to the abdominal wall (Fig. 5).

> **TIP**
>
> *Pneumoperitoneum is established with an intra-abdominal pressure higher than 10 mmHg.*

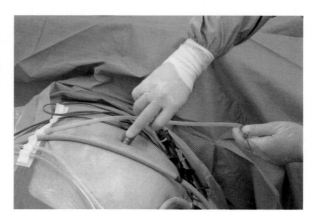

FIG. 5

Perpendicular introduction of the trocar

The optic is introduced through the trocar, and the abdomen is then inspected for any injury due to insertion of the Veress needle or the trocar, and to identify adhesions in areas where the secondary ports will be placed.

> **TIP**
>
> *After trocar placement and obturator removal, the trocar valve is briefly opened to check for egress of gas, confirming it is correctly placed inside the abdomen. The insufflator line is then connected to the trocar.*

Second Port (5 mm, monopolar round-tipped scissors)

The triangulation rule must be followed for the placement of the trocars as the body habitus is different for each patient: *four fingerbreadths between the optic trocar and the working trocars* (Fig. 6), and *five fingerbreadths between the working trocars* (Fig. 7a,b).

> **TIP**
>
> *To prevent lens fogging, insert the distal end of the optic into warm sterile water or saline before intra-abdominal optic introduction.*

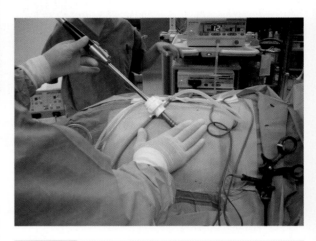

FIG. 6

Triangulation rule, four fingers

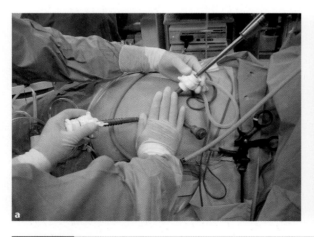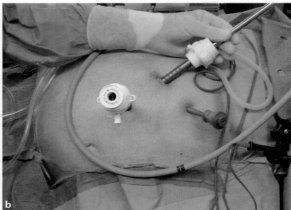

FIG. 7

a Triangulation rule, five fingers. **b** Ports in place

TIP

The 5-mm port is usually reserved for the most skilled hand, as the movements of the working instruments must be more precise inside the smaller ports.

Third Port (11 mm, bipolar grasper)

The triangulation rule must be followed as above.

Fourth Port (5 mm, suction device)

For the introduction of the 5-mm trocar, a cutaneous incision is made approximately midline between the umbilicus trocar and the anterior superior iliac spine on the side of the procedure.

Fifth Port (5 mm, liver retractor grasper)

If liver retraction is necessary during a right-side nephrectomy, a cutaneous incision is made approximately two fingerbreadths below the level of the second port, and a 5-mm port is introduced (Fig. 8).

Final Position of the Ports (see Figs. 8 and 9)

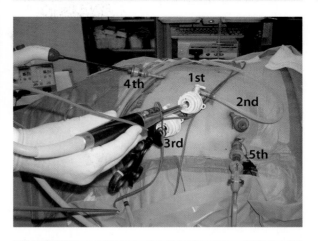

FIG. 8
Right-side ports

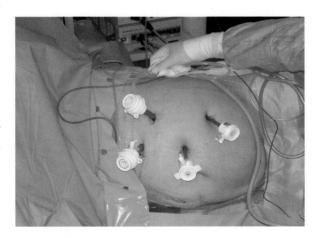

FIG. 9
Left-side ports

Surgical Technique

Colon Mobilization

For a *left-side nephrectomy*, the plane between the descending colon and the underlying Gerota's fascia is developed to allow the colon to fall medially (Fig. 10a–c).

TIP

The lateral attachments of Gerota's fascia to the abdominal wall should not be freed at this time to avoid the kidney falling medially into the operating field.

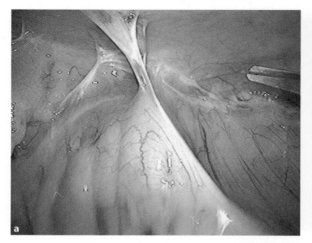

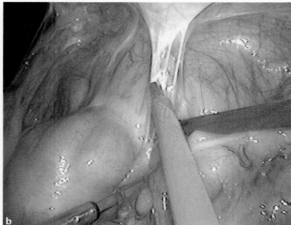

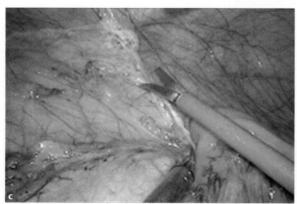

FIG. 10

a Colon attachments to abdominal wall. **b** Release of colon attachments to abdominal wall. **c** Colon is dissected from Gerota's fascia (Gerota is not freed from abdominal wall)

This plane of dissection is carried out cranially. The splenorenal and lienocolic ligaments are incised, allowing the spleen and the tail of the pancreas to be separated from the upper pole of the kidney. The en bloc dissection of the colon, spleen, and pancreas must be completed for adequate exposure of the renal vein (Fig. 11a,b).

For a *right-side nephrectomy*, the liver is cranially retracted using a grasper that is fixed to the abdominal wall (Fig. 12). The ascending colon is mobilized and dissected from the underlying Gerota's fascia. Mobilization of the colon continues caudally to the common iliac vessels.

Ureter and Gonadal Vessels Identification

Following the medial mobilization of the colon and mesocolon, the gonadal vessels are visualized. After the colon is medially retracted, the Gerota's fatty tissue at the level of the lower pole of the kidney is incised and lifted to locate the psoas muscle (Fig. 13).

> **TIP**
>
> *The correct maneuver to expose the psoas muscle is the continuous upper movement of the laparoscopic instruments to lift the fatty tissue.*

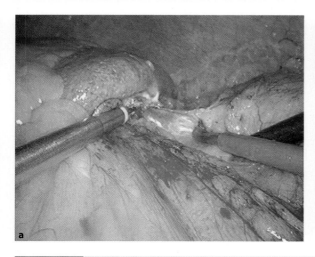

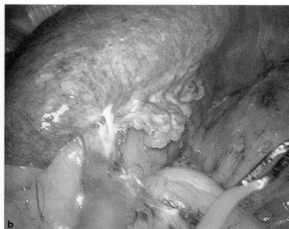

FIG. 11

a Spleen is released from kidney. **b** En bloc spleen dissection

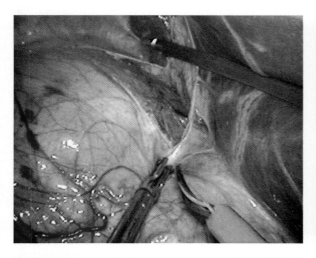

FIG. 12

Grasper retracting liver

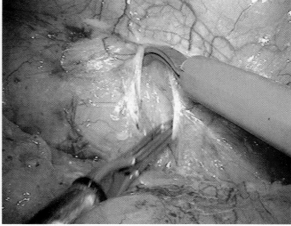

FIG. 13

Lifting of fatty tissue to expose psoas muscle

The psoas is followed to expose the ureter just lateral and deep to the gonadal vessels.

Caudally, the ureter is dissected and freed until the crossing of the iliac vessels. The ureter and gonadal ves-sels are not divided at this time. Both structures are lifted and, by visualization of the psoas muscle (Fig. 14a,b), followed cranially to the lower pole and hilum of the kidney (Fig. 15a,b).

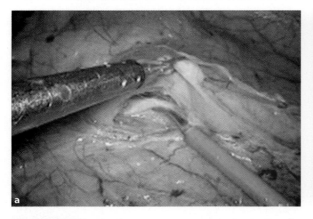

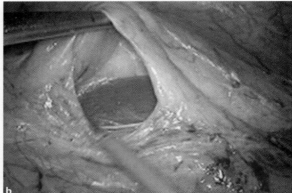

FIG. 14

a Dissection of ureter and gonadal vessels. **b** Psoas muscle

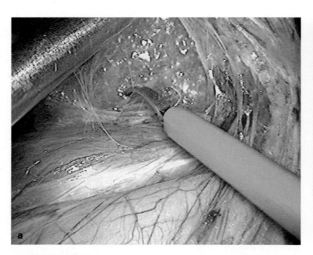

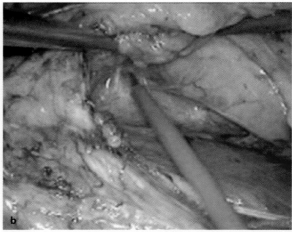

FIG. 15

a Psoas is followed cranially to hilum. **b** Ureter and gonadal vessels approaching renal hilum

The dissection of the right gonadal vein is not necessary, as it enters the vena cava on this side. Attachments between the psoas muscle and Gerota's fascia are released by sharp and blunt dissection, and small vessels to the ureter and branches of the gonadal vein are coagulated with the bipolar grasper.

Exposure and Dissection of the Renal Hilum

On the left, tracking the course of the left gonadal vein into the renal vein and firm elevation of the lower pole of the kidney on both sides assists in the identification and blunt dissection of the renal hilum.

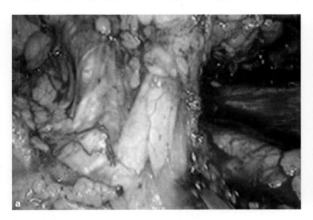

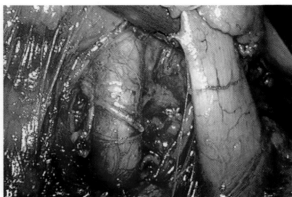

FIG. 16

a Renal hilum exposed. **b** Dissection of renal vessels

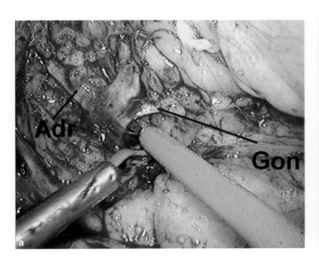

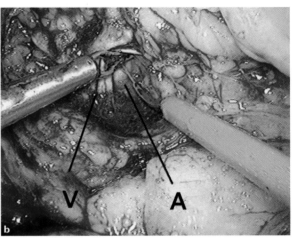

FIG. 17

a Left adrenal vein (Adr); Gonadal vein (Gon). **b** Renal vein (V); Renal artery (A)

The renal vessels should be individually dissected (Fig. 16a,b).

The renal vein is dissected, taking care with the lumbar veins that drain posterior to the vessel (Fig. 17a,b). The left adrenal vein is preserved if the ipsilateral adrenal gland is not removed.

TIP

Dissection of the right renal vein is usually less demanding as lumbar veins are normally absent at this side.

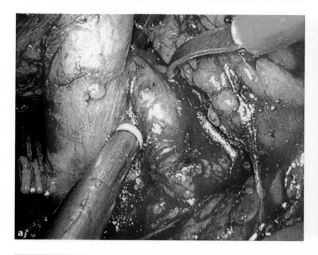 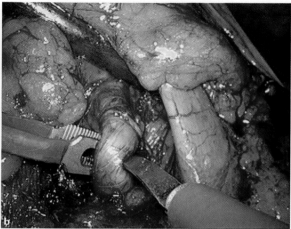

FIG. 18

a Renal artery posterior to renal vein. **b** Dissection of the renal artery

The renal artery is exposed posterior to the renal vein and dissected (Fig. 18a,b).

Renal Hilum Ligature and Transection

Hem-o-lok® polymer clips (Weck, Teleflex Medical) are applied to the artery.

> **TIP**
>
> *One extra-large (XL) clip secures the renal artery before the renal vein is clipped.*

Three clips (XL Hem-o-lok) are used on the renal vein, which is then carefully transected.

> **TIP**
>
> *The renal vein should be flat after the renal artery clip is placed; if the vein is still filling, another renal artery should be located.*

Following division of the renal vein, clipping of the renal artery is completed (3 XL Hem-o-lok clips), and the vessel is then transected.

Mobilization of the Kidney and Adrenal Gland

Once all the hilar vessels have been divided, the dissection continues posteriorly and superiorly to the upper pole. The attachments of the kidney to the posterior and lateral abdominal wall are released by blunt and sharp dissection, taking care to coagulate the bleeding vessels. The adrenal gland can be preserved in a simple nephrectomy and particular cases of mid- and lower-pole tumors, but otherwise are removed intact with the specimen. This is accomplished by incising Gerota's fascia anteriorly just above the hilum (Fig. 19). Gerota's fascia is then gently peeled off circumferentially above the upper pole of the kidney. At this point during the dissection, care must be taken with the short adrenal vein on the right side that drains posterolateral into the vena cava. On the right, superior retraction of the liver facilitates the dissection of the plane between the liver and the upper pole of the kidney (Fig. 20).

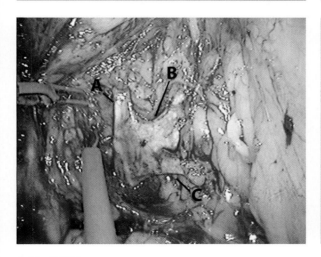

FIG. 19
Left adrenal vein (A); Left renal vein (B); Gonadal vein (C)

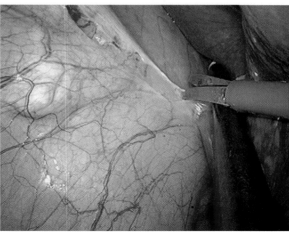

FIG. 20
Plane between kidney and liver

Transection of the Ureter

Inferiorly, the ureter is double-clipped with (L) Hem-o-lok® clips and transected to allow the kidney to be fully mobilized. This facilitates the dissection and incision of the lateroposterior and uppermost attachments under direct vision.

> **TIP**
>
> *Both ureteral ends are clipped to avoid urine spillage in case a transitional cell carcinoma is present.*

Kidney Extraction

A lower ilioinguinal muscle-splitting incision (Gibson type) is performed, but the muscle attached to the peritoneum is not incised. A large laparoscopic bag *(Endo Catch® II 15 mm, Tyco Autosuture)* is introduced through the small opening of the ilioinguinal incision.

The kidney is placed intact inside the bag and the specimen is removed.

> **TIP**
>
> *The string of the bag is pulled out to close it, and the arm of the device is retracted to liberate the metal ring.*

Closure of the Abdominal Wall

The abdominal wall is closed using running Vicryl 2-0 SH 1 Plus (needle ½ 21.8 mm) for the peritoneum, Vicryl 0 suture in "X" for the muscle, and running Vicryl 1 CT Plus (needle ½ 39.9 mm) for the aponeurosis. Once the abdominal wall is closed, pneumoperitoneum is re-established and the optic introduced for revision of the hemostasis. A silicone Penrose drain is inserted. After evacuation of the pneumoperitoneum and removal of the trocars, the aponeurosis of the 11-mm ports is closed with a Dexon™ II HGU-46 suture. The skin incisions are closed with subcuticular Monocryl® 3-0 C 423.

Postoperative Considerations

The nasogastric tube is removed at the end of the procedure, and the intravenous perfusion is stopped on day 1. Pain is controlled with scheduled intramuscular nonsteroidal anti-inflammatory drugs (NSAIDs) and oral analgesics. Intramuscular NSAIDs are often discontinued after 24 hours. A light diet can generally be resumed one day after surgery. The Foley catheter is usually removed on day 1 and the Penrose drain on day 2 after surgery. The patient leaves the hospital on the third or fourth postoperative day. Patients can resume normal light activities after hospital discharge, but vigorous activities and heavy lifting are limited for at least one month after surgery.

Suggested Readings

1. Hemal AK, Kumar A: Laparoscopic versus open radical nephrectomy for large renal tumors: a long-term prospective comparison. J Urol 2007 Mar; 177(3):862–866.
2. Mattar K, Finelli A: Expanding the indications for laparoscopic radical nephrectomy. Curr Opin Urol 2007 Mar; 17(2):88–92.
3. Kouba E, Smith AM: Efficacy and safety of en bloc ligation of renal hilum during laparoscopic nephrectomy. Urology 2007 Feb; 69(2):226–229.
4. Permpongkosol S, Link RE: Complications of 2,775 urological laparoscopic procedures: 1993 to 2005. J Urol 2007 Feb; 177(2):580–585.
5. Gong EM, Lyon MB: Laparoscopic radical nephrectomy: comparison of clinical Stage T1 and T2 renal tumors. Urology 2006 Dec; 68(6):1183–1187.
6. Romero FR, Muntener M: Pure laparoscopic radical nephrectomy with level II vena caval thrombectomy. Urology 2006 Nov; 68(5):1112–1114.
7. Ono Y, Hattori R: Laparoscopic radical nephrectomy for renal cell carcinoma: the standard of care already? Curr Opin Urol. 2005 Mar; 15(2):75–78.

Chapter 3

Transperitoneal Laparoscopic Partial Nephrectomy

Contents

Introduction

Since the introduction of cross-sectional imaging for the diagnosis of intra-abdominal pathologies, an increased number of small renal masses are being incidentally discovered. These lesions are often peripherally located, with a benign histology in less than half of the cases. Following removal, no significant differences in survival rates exist between patients who have undergone partial or radical nephrectomy. In addition, the local recurrence rate after nephron-sparing surgery (NSS) is less than 3%. For all of these reasons, and motivated by the benefits of decreased patient morbidity and fast recovery, laparoscopic partial nephrectomy is successfully becoming the standard of care for the surgical management of exophytic renal tumors 4 cm in diameter or smaller. However, despite the potential advantages of nephron-sparing surgery and the laparoscopic approach over open surgery, laparoscopic partial nephrectomy is still not widely performed because of technical difficulties inherent to the procedure. There is ongoing debate regarding the need for complete hilar clamping, warm ischemia time, and the use of haemostatic techniques after tumor removal. Even in skilled hands, this complex procedure is still evolving. The technique described uses a transperitoneal route and an extracorporeal clamp approach of delayed occlusion and early release of the renal pedicle to minimize warm ischemia time.

Preoperative Preparation

Before a patient consents to a laparoscopic partial nephrectomy, it is important to discuss the specific risks of the surgery, including the potential need to convert to the traditional open operation if difficulties arise.

The patient is admitted to the hospital the night before the surgery for bowel preparation, which includes 2 L of Colopeg® (1 envelope/L) p.o. and a Fleet® enema. Fasting starts at midnight before surgery. Thromboprophylaxis protocol is implemented with good hydration, placement of compressive elastic stockings on the lower extremities, and low-molecular-weight heparin. Enoxaparin (Clexane®, Lovenox®) 40 mg sc 1 × day or nadroparin (Flaxiparine®, Fraxiparin®) 0.6 mL sc 1 × day is initiated on day 1 after the surgery and continued daily until the patient is discharged from the hospital. In selected cases, the treatment is continued for 30 days after the procedure. Patients also receive antibiotic prophylaxis with a single preoperative dose of intravenous second-generation cephalosporin, unless they are allergic to penicillin. Blood type and crossmatch are determined.

Patient Positioning and Initial Preparation

The patient is initially positioned supine for IV access, the induction of general anesthesia, and endotracheal intubation. An orogastric tube is placed and the stomach decompressed to avoid puncture during trocar placement and to allow additional space during abdominal insufflation. An 18Fr Foley catheter with 10 mL in the balloon is introduced for decompression of the bladder. During skin preparation, the entire flank and abdomen are included in case conversion to an open procedure is required. The umbilicus is placed over the break in the operating table, and the patient is positioned in a modified lateral decubitus position.

> **TIP**
>
> *For a left-side nephrectomy, the patient is placed in a strict lateral decubitus position.*

The table can be flexed as needed, or an inflatable balloon is positioned under the patient at the level of the umbilicus. Padding is used to support the buttocks and dorsum, and all potential pressure points are cushioned. An axillary roll is placed to prevent brachial plexus injury, and the arms should be positioned as far away from the trunk as possible so as not to disturb the movement of the operative team. The patient is held in position with strips of cloth tape (Fig. 1a,b).

The surgeon operates from the abdominal side of the

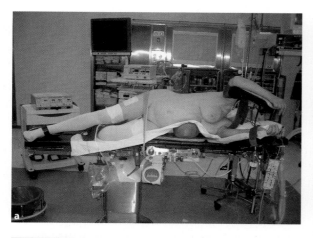
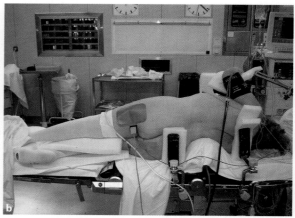

FIG. 1

a Patient position. b Padding

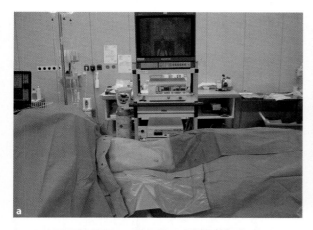

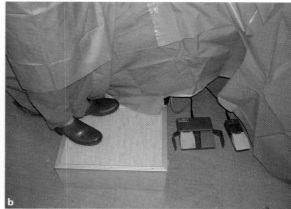

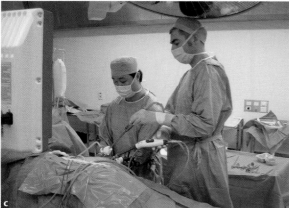

FIG. 2

a Patient and laparoscopic cart. **b** Steps below assistant.
c Instruments table behind operative team

patient, and the first assistant is placed caudally to the surgeon. The laparoscopic cart is positioned at the back of the patient's chest with the operative team facing the video monitor. The instruments table is positioned behind the operative team, and the assistant is positioned higher than the surgeon to prevent laparoscopic instruments from conflicting (Fig. 2a–c).

Trocars and Laparoscopic Instruments

- 3 × 11 mm (optic 0°, Satinsky vascular clamp, and bipolar grasper)
- 3 × 5 mm for right-side partial nephrectomy (scissors, suction device, and liver retractor grasper)

- 2 × 5 mm for left-side partial nephrectomy (scissors and suction device)
- Monopolar round-tipped scissors, bipolar grasper, Satinsky vascular clamp, liver retractor grasper, 5-mm suction device, needle drivers (2), and 10-mm laparoscopic optic 0°

Access and Port Placement

Five ports are generally enough to perform the procedure, although a sixth trocar may be necessary for liver retraction during a right-side partial nephrectomy (Fig. 3). Before trocars are placed, the abdomen is insufflated using a Veress needle.

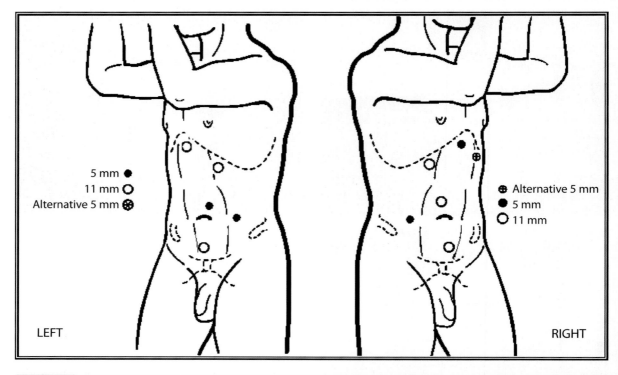

5 mm ●
11 mm ○
Alternative 5 mm ✸

⊕ Alternative 5 mm
● 5 mm
○ 11 mm

LEFT   RIGHT

FIG. 3

Access and port placement (This figure was published in Wein: Campbell-Walsh Urology, 9th ed., Copyright Elsevier)

> **TIP**
>
> *In case of previous surgery, the Veress needle is not inserted, and the open access technique is used to place the first trocar.*

> **TIP**
>
> *The skin incision should be 50% larger than the diameter of the 11-mm trocar.*

The Veress needle is introduced through the incision (see Chap. 1, Veress Needle Introduction).

Veress Needle

A cutaneous incision is made two fingerbreadths below the costal margin arch in the midaxillary line, lateral to the ipsilateral rectus muscle (Fig. 4a,b).

First Port (11 mm, optic 0°)

Once pneumoperitoneum is established, the Veress needle is removed, and the 11-mm trocar is introduced through the same incision, perpendicularly to the abdominal wall (Fig. 5).

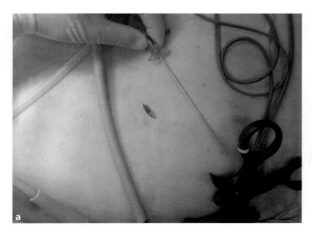

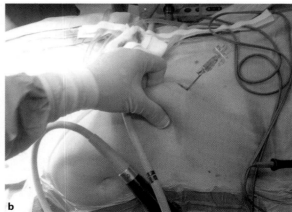

FIG. 4
a Cutaneous incision below costal margin. **b** Insertion of Veress needle

---

> **TIP**
>
> *Pneumoperitoneum is established with an intra-abdominal pressure higher than 10 mmHg.*

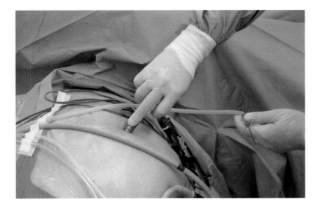

FIG. 5
Perpendicular introduction of the trocar

The optic is introduced through the trocar, and the abdomen is then inspected for any injury due to insertion of the Veress needle or the trocar, and to identify adhesions in areas where the secondary ports will be placed.

> **TIP**
>
> *After trocar placement and obturator removal, the trocar valve is briefly opened to check for egress of gas, confirming it is correctly placed inside the abdomen. The insufflator line is then connected to the trocar.*

Second Port
(5 mm, monopolar round-tipped scissors)

The triangulation rule must be followed for the placement of the trocars as the body habitus is different for each patient: *four fingerbreadths between the optic trocar and the working trocars* (Fig. 6), and *five fingerbreadths between the working trocars* (Fig. 7a,b).

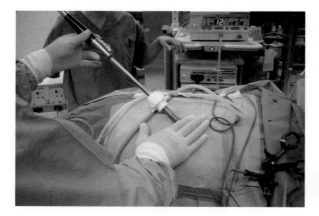

FIG. 6

Triangulation rule, four fingers

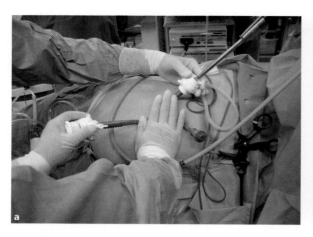
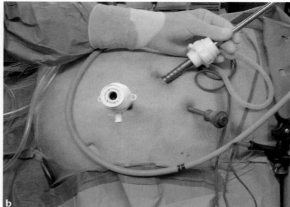

FIG. 7

a Triangulation rule, five fingers. **b** Ports in place

TIP

The skin incision should be 50% larger than the diameter of the trocar.

Third Port (11 mm, bipolar grasper)

The triangulation rule must be followed as above.

Fourth Port (5 mm, suction device)

For the introduction of the 5-mm trocar, a cutaneous incision is made approximately midline between the umbilicus trocar and the anterior superior iliac spine on the side of the procedure.

Fifth Port (5 mm, liver retractor grasper)

If liver retraction is necessary during a right-side partial nephrectomy, a cutaneous incision is made approxi-

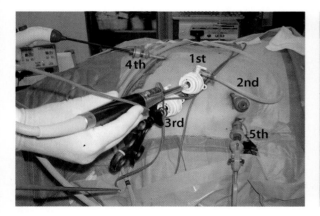

FIG. 8
Right-side ports

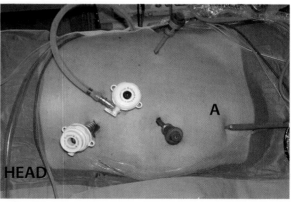

FIG. 9
11-mm port for introduction of Satinsky vascular clamp (A)

mately two fingerbreadths below the level of the second port, and a 5-mm port is introduced (Fig. 8).

Sixth Port (11 mm, Satinsky vascular clamp)

A cutaneous incision is made approximately in line with the most caudal trocar but placed slightly inferior to the umbilicus (Fig. 9).

> **TIP**
>
> *The 11-mm trocar for the Satinsky vascular clamp is inserted only after the exposure and dissection of the renal hilum.*

Final Position of the Ports

The ports are tied to the skin with Vicryl® 2-0 to prevent accidental removal.

Surgical Technique

Colon Mobilization

For a left-side partial nephrectomy, the plane between the descending colon and the underlying Gerota's fascia is developed to allow the colon to fall medially (Fig. 10a–c).

> **TIP**
>
> *The lateral attachments of the kidney to the abdominal wall should not be freed at this time to avoid the kidney falling medially into the operating field.*

This plane of dissection is carried out cranially. The splenorenal and lienocolic ligaments are incised, allowing the spleen and the tail of the pancreas to be separated from the upper pole of the kidney (Fig. 11a,b).

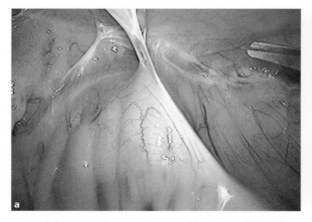

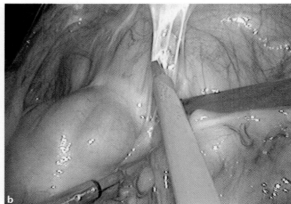

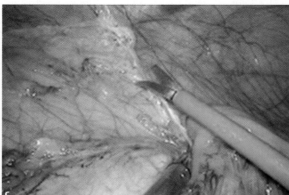

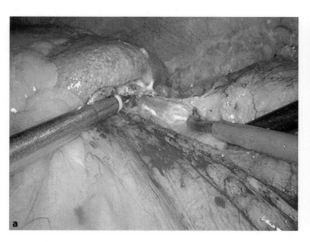

FIG. 10

a Colon attachments to abdominal wall. **b** Release of colon attachments to abdominal wall. **c** Colon is dissected from Gerota's fascia (Gerota is not freed from abdominal wall)

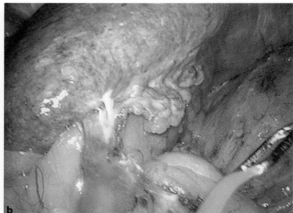

FIG. 11

a Spleen is released from kidney. **b** En bloc spleen dissection

TIP

In this maneuver, the weight of the spleen dissected en bloc opens the space spontaneously.

For a right-side partial nephrectomy, the liver is cranially retracted using a grasper that is fixed to the abdominal wall (Fig. 12).

The ascending colon is mobilized and dissected from the underlying Gerota's fascia. Colon mobilization continues caudally to the common iliac vessels to expose the lower pole of the kidney, the ureter, and the gonadal vessels.

Ureter and Gonadal Vessels Identification

After the colon is medially retracted, the Gerota's fatty tissue at the level of the lower pole of the kidney is incised and lifted to locate the psoas muscle (Fig. 13).

TIP

The correct maneuver to expose the psoas muscle is the continuous upper movement of the laparoscopic instruments to lift the fatty tissue.

The psoas is followed to expose the gonadal vessels and the ureter just lateral and deep to these vessels. Both structures are elevated and, by visualization of the psoas muscle (Fig. 14a,b), followed cranially to the lower pole and hilum of the kidney.

Attachments between the psoas muscle and Gerota's fascia are released with sharp and blunt dissection, and small vessels to the ureter and branches of the gonadal vein are coagulated with the bipolar grasper.

Exposure and Dissection of the Renal Hilum

On the left, tracking the course of the left gonadal vein into the renal vein and firm elevation of the lower pole of the kidney on both sides assists in the identification and blunt dissection of the renal hilum (Fig. 15).

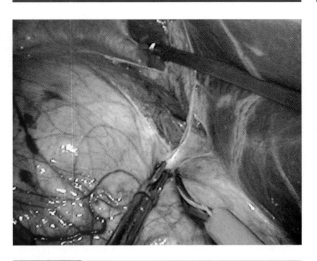

FIG. 12
Grasper retracting liver

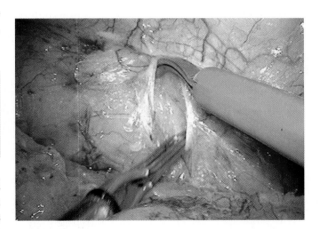

FIG. 13
Lifting of fatty tissue to expose psoas muscle

The renal vein is dissected, taking care with the lumbar veins that drain posterior to the vessel. The renal artery is routinely not dissected. The Satinsky vascular clamp is introduced and positioned around the pedicle, but it is not clamped at this time (Figs. 9 and 16a,b).

The renal vessels should be clamped en bloc, but a single vein is left unclamped to permit venous drainage in case an accessory renal artery was missed and not properly secured (Fig. 17a,b).

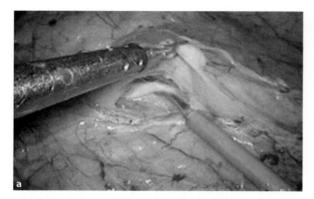

TIP

The en bloc clamping of the pedicle using a large Satinsky clamp is technically faster as less dissection is required, but there is always a risk of parenchymal flow overpressure due to a missed polar artery, which can jeopardize bleeding control. For this reason, it is safer to completely dissect the kidney to exclude an accessory artery when performing the en bloc hilar control.

Localization of the Kidney Tumor

The Gerota's fascia overlying the area where the tumor is likely to be found is incised with monopolar scissors (Fig. 18). Palpation with the tip of the instrument also aids in this objective.

Tumor Resection

The fatty tissue overlying the tumor is removed and sent to pathology. The surface of the renal cortex bordering the lesion is stripped of fatty tissue to permit good visualization of the lateral margins of the tumor (Fig. 19).

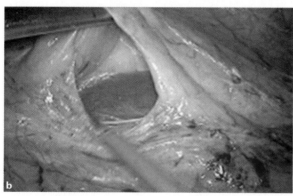

FIG. 14

a Dissection of ureter and gonadal vessels. b Psoas muscle

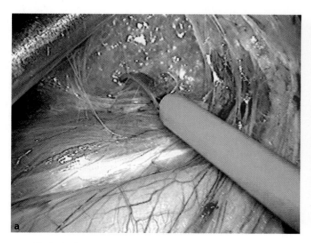

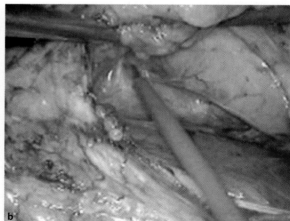

FIG. 15

a Psoas is followed cranially to hilum. b Ureter and gonadal vessels approaching renal hilum

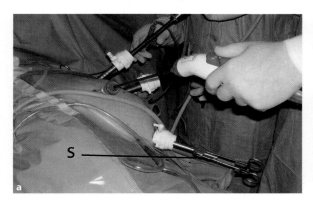
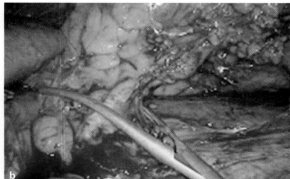

FIG. 16
a Satinsky vascular clamp (S). **b** Satinsky around the pedicle

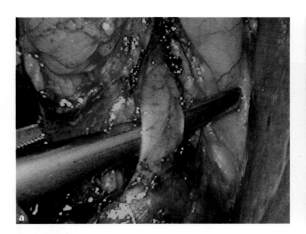
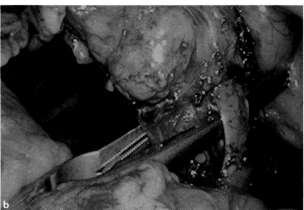

FIG. 17
a Satinsky vascular clamp around the hilum. **b** Renal vein left unclamped

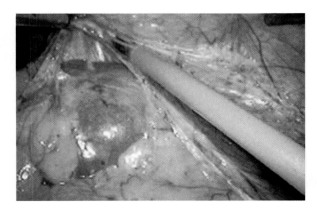

FIG. 18
Gerota's fascia incised over tumor

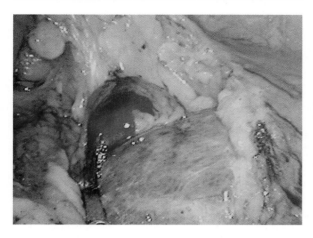

FIG. 19

Renal cortex surface around nodule stripped of fatty tissue

The Gerota's fascia is mobilized beyond the margins of the wedge resection to facilitate posterior kidney reconstruction. After delimitating a tumor-free margin of at least 0.5 cm, the cortex and renal parenchyma around the nodule are incised with monopolar scissors. At this time, if necessary, the pedicle is clamped and the ischemia time begins. The renal parenchyma bordering the nodule is coagulated and cut with the same instrument, and the tumor is completely excised (Fig. 20a–c).

If a renal calyx is opened during the resection, a running suture of Vicryl 2-0 is used to close the defect following tumor removal (Fig. 21a,b).

Interrupted U-shaped sutures of Vicryl 0 GS 24 are placed through the Gerota and the renal parenchyma (Fig. 22).

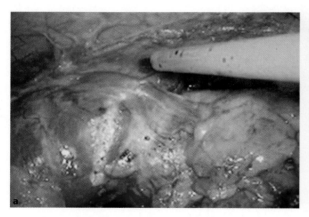

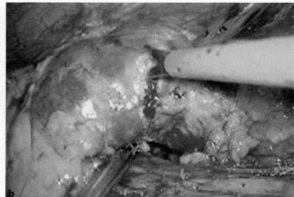

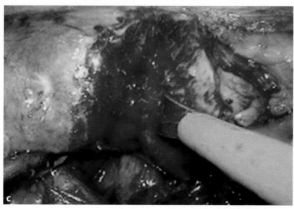

FIG. 20

a Demarcation of the incision. **b** Renal parenchyma is cut.
c Tumor excision

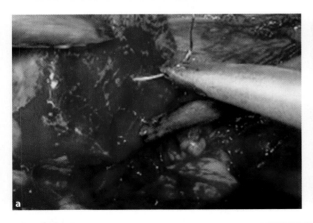
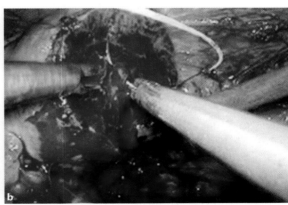

FIG. 21

a Open calyx. **b** Suture closing open calyx

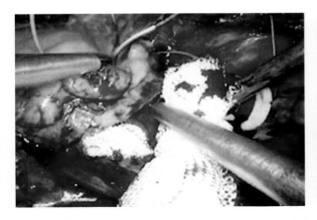
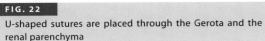

FIG. 22

U-shaped sutures are placed through the Gerota and the renal parenchyma

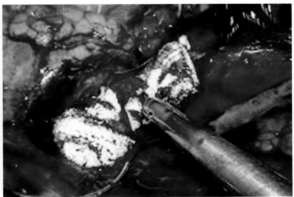

FIG. 23

Surgical bolsters

Two Surgicel® bolsters 10 × 20 cm are placed under the loose loops of the suture to fill in the defect and help with the hemostasis (Fig. 23).

The knot is gently and carefully tied to avoid tearing of the parenchyma. The vascular clamp is opened, and any eventual bleeding is controlled with a further Vicryl 0 suture (Fig. 24).

Closure of the Abdominal Wall

The specimen is placed in an Endo Catch® bag (Tyco Autosuture), and the incision is enlarged for specimen removal. A 12-mm silicone Penrose drain is introduced. The aponeurosis of the 11-mm ports is closed with a Dexon™ II HGU-46 suture, and the skin incisions are

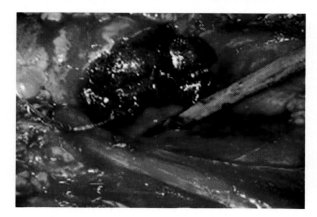

FIG. 24
Final result

closed with running intradermic Monocryl® 3-0. The Penrose is sutured to the skin with Flexidene® 2-0, and the skin incision is closed with an Opsite® dressing.

Postoperative Considerations

The nasogastric tube is removed at the end of the procedure, and the intravenous perfusion is stopped on day 1. Pain is controlled with scheduled intramuscular non-steroidal anti-inflammatory drugs (NSAIDs) and oral analgesics. Intramuscular NSAIDs are often discontinued after 24 h. A light diet can generally be resumed

on day 1 after surgery. The Foley catheter is usually removed on the first post-operative day, and the Penrose drain is removed before discharge or when drainage is less than 50 mL. Patients can resume normal light activities after hospital discharge, but vigorous activities and heavy lifting are limited for at least one month after surgery.

Suggested Readings

1. Orvieto MA, Zorn KC: Recovery of renal function after complete renal hilar versus artery alone clamping during open and laparoscopic surgery. J Urol 2007 Jun; 177(6):2371–2374.

2. Verhoest G, Manunta A: Laparoscopic partial nephrectomy with clamping of the renal parenchyma: initial experience. Eur Urol 2007 Nov; 52(5):1340–6.

3. Bollens R, Rosenblatt A: Laparoscopic partial nephrectomy with "on-demand" clamping reduces warm ischemia time. Eur Urol 2007 Apr; 52(3): 804–810.

4. Van Dijk JH, Pes PL: Haemostasis in laparoscopic partial nephrectomy: current status. Minim Invasive Ther Allied Technol 2007; 16(1):31–44.

5. Häcker A, Albadour A: Nephron-sparing surgery for renal tumours: acceleration and facilitation of the laparoscopic technique. Eur Urol 2007 Feb; 51(2):358–365.

6. Breda A, Stepanian SV: Use of haemostatic agents and glues during laparoscopic partial nephrectomy: a multi-institutional survey from the United States and Europe of 1347 cases. Eur Urol 2007 Feb; 52(3):798–803.

Laparoscopic Assisted Transperitoneal Nephroureterectomy

Contents

Introduction

In recent years, laparoscopic nephroureterectomy has been developed and applied to patients with transitional cell carcinoma (TCC) of the renal pelvis and ureter. The laparoscopic approach results in less blood loss, fewer postoperative pain and analgesic requirements, and faster recovery to normal activity compared with open nephroureterectomy. The main issue of this procedure is the oncologic control, particularly the management of the distal ureter. The en bloc ureteral resection to avoid tumor spillage is the preferred method, and many innovative techniques have been used to address the subject.

With the technique here described, the kidney and proximal ureter are dissected laparoscopically by way of a transperitoneal approach, and an ilioinguinal incision (Gibson-type) is performed for continued dissection of the distal ureter with a cuff of bladder. The abdominal incision permits safe specimen removal, reducing the technical complexity of the procedure and operative times.

Preoperative Preparation

Before a patient consents to a laparoscopic nephroureterectomy, it is important to discuss the specific risks of the surgery, including the potential need to convert to the traditional open operation if difficulties arise.

The patient is admitted to the hospital the day before the surgery for bowel preparation, which includes 2 L of Colopeg® (1 envelope/L) p.o. and a Fleet® enema. Fasting starts at midnight before surgery. Thromboprophylaxis protocol is implemented with good hydration, placement of compressive elastic stockings on the lower extremities, and low-molecular-weight heparin. Enoxaparin (Clexane®, Lovenox®) 40 mg sc 1 × day or nadroparin (Flaxiparine®, Fraxiparin®) 0.6 mL sc 1 × day is initiated on day 1 after the surgery and continued daily until the patient is discharged from the hospital. In selected cases, the treatment is continued for 30 days after the procedure. Patients also receive antibiotic prophylaxis with a single preoperative dose of intravenous second-generation cephalosporin, unless they are allergic to penicillin. Blood type and crossmatch are determined.

Patient Positioning and Initial Preparation

The patient is initially positioned supine for intravenous access, the induction of general anesthesia, and endotracheal intubation. An orogastric tube is placed and the stomach decompressed to avoid puncture during trocar placement and to allow additional space during abdominal insufflation. An 18Fr Foley catheter with 10 mL in the balloon is introduced for bladder decompression. During skin preparation, the entire flank and abdomen are included in case conversion to an open procedure is required. The umbilicus is placed over the break in the operating table, and the patient is positioned in a modified lateral decubitus position.

> **TIP**
>
> *For a left-side nephroureterectomy, the patient is placed in a strict lateral decubitus position.*

The table can be flexed as needed, or an inflatable balloon is positioned under the patient at the level of the umbilicus. Padding is used to support the buttocks and dorsum, and all potential pressure points are cushioned. An axillary roll is placed to prevent brachial plexus injury, and the arms should be positioned as far away from the trunk as possible so as not to disturb the movement of the operative team. The patient is held in position with strips of cloth tape (Fig. 1a,b).

The surgeon operates from the abdominal side of the patient, and the first assistant is placed caudally to the surgeon. The laparoscopic cart is positioned at the back of the patient's chest with the operative team facing the video monitor. The instruments table is positioned

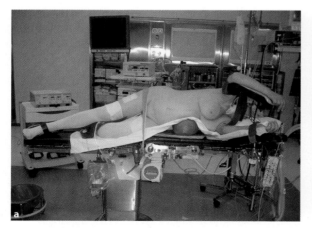 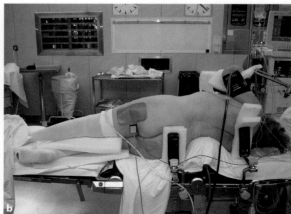

FIG. 1

a Patient's position. **b** Padding

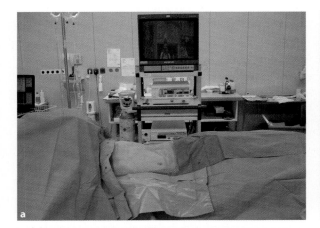

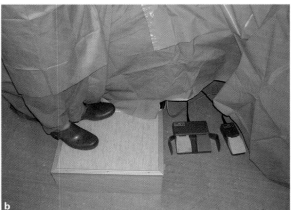

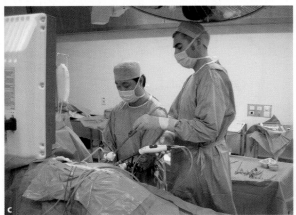

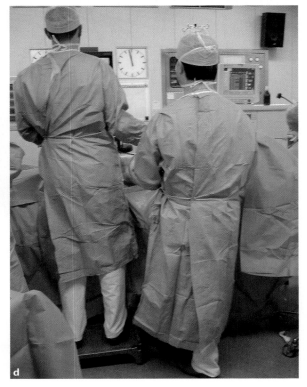

FIG. 2

a Patient and laparoscopic cart. **b** Steps below assistant. **c** Instruments table behind operative team. **d** Operative team's position

behind the operative team, and the assistant stands on steps (Fig. 2a–d).

Trocars and Laparoscopic Instruments

Right-side nephroureterectomy:
- 2 × 11 mm (optic 0°, bipolar grasper, 10 mm-clip applier)
- 3 × 5 mm (monopolar scissors, suction device, and liver retractor grasper)

Left-side nephroureterectomy:
- 2 × 11 mm (optic 0° and bipolar grasper)
- 2 × 5 mm (scissors and suction device)

- Monopolar round-tipped scissors, bipolar grasper, liver retractor grasper, 5-mm suction device, Ethicon 10-mm clip applier (non-disposable), needle drivers (2), and 10-mm laparoscopic optic 0°

Access and Port Placement

Four ports are generally sufficient to complete the procedure, although a fifth trocar may be necessary for liver retraction during a right-side nephroureterectomy (Fig. 3).

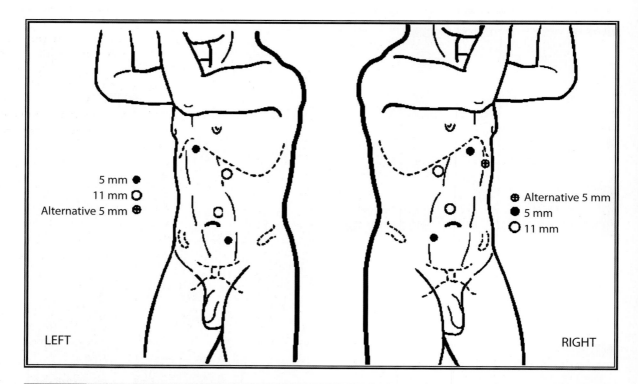

5 mm ●
11 mm ○
Alternative 5 mm ⊕

⊕ Alternative 5 mm
● 5 mm
○ 11 mm

LEFT

RIGHT

FIG. 3

Access and port placement (This figure was published in Wein: Campbell-Walsh Urology, 9th ed., Copyright Elsevier)

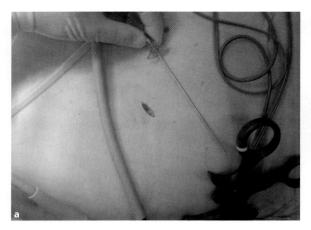

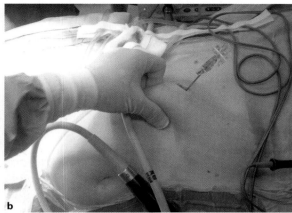

FIG. 4

a Cutaneous incision below costal margin. **b** Insertion of Veress needle

Veress Needle

A cutaneous incision is made two fingerbreadths below the costal margin arch, at the level of the lateral border of the rectus muscle (Fig. 4a,b).

> **TIP**
>
> *The skin incision should be 50% larger than the diameter of the 11-mm trocar.*

The Veress needle is introduced through the incision (see Chap. 1, Veress Needle Introduction).

First Port (11 mm, optic 0°)

Once pneumoperitoneum is established, the needle is removed, and the 11-mm trocar is introduced through the same incision, perpendicularly to the abdominal wall (Fig. 5).

> **TIP**
>
> *Pneumoperitoneum is established with an intra-abdominal pressure higher than 10 mmHg.*

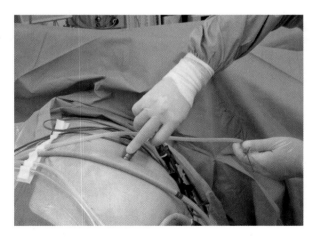

FIG. 5

Perpendicular introduction of the trocar

The optic is introduced through the trocar, and the abdomen is then inspected for any injury due to insertion of the Veress needle or the trocar, and to identify adhesions in areas where the secondary ports will be placed.

Second Port

- For a right-side nephroureterectomy: 5 mm (monopolar round-tipped scissors)
- For a left-side nephroureterectomy: 11 mm – positioned around the umbilicus (monopolar round-tipped scissors, optic, 10-mm clip applier)

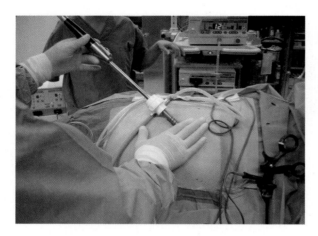

FIG. 6
Triangulation rule for right-side nephroureterectomy

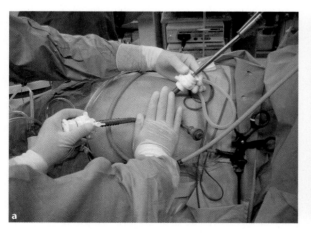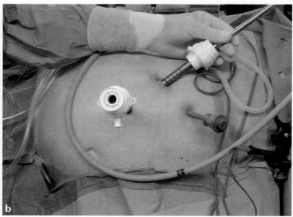

FIG. 7
a Triangulation rule. **b** Ports in place

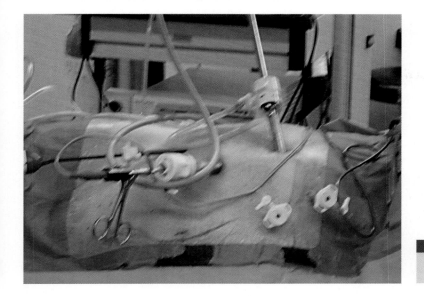

FIG. 8

Fourth port (caudal port) in line with the periumbilical port

TIP

The position of the working trocars for a left-side nephroureterectomy are switched over when compared to the transperitoneal laparoscopic nephrectomy; therefore, the 5-mm port is placed at the xiphoid process, and the 11-mm port is placed close to the umbilicus (see Chap. 2, Access and Port Placement).

The triangulation rule must be followed for the placement of the trocars as the body habitus is different for each patient: four fingerbreadths between the optic trocar and the working trocars (Fig. 6), and five fingerbreadths between the working trocars (Fig. 7a,b).

Third Port

- For a left-side nephroureterectomy: 5 mm positioned at the xiphoid process (bipolar grasper)
- For a right-side nephroureterectomy: 11 mm (bipolar grasper, optic)
  The triangulation rule must be followed as above.

Fourth Port (5 mm, suction device)

For the introduction of the 5-mm trocar, a cutaneous incision is made approximately three fingers caudally to the umbilicus and in line with the periumbilical trocar (Fig. 8).

TIP

This trocar is positioned lower than for the transperitoneal laparoscopic nephrectomy; the trocar will be used for the placement of a bipolar grasper during the ureteral part of the procedure (Fig. 9).

Fifth Port (5 mm, liver retractor grasper)

If liver retraction is necessary during a right-side nephroureterectomy, a cutaneous incision is made approximately two fingerbreadths below the level of the second port, and a 5-mm trocar is introduced.

The ports are finally tied to the skin with Vicryl® 2-0 to prevent accidental removal.

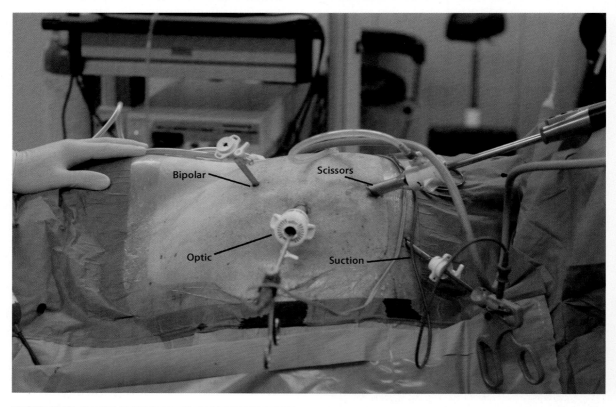

FIG. 9

Reposition of the instruments (see Access for the lower ureteral dissection)

Access for the Lower Ureteral Dissection

During the ureteral part of the procedure, the position of the instruments is changed for the ureteral dissection. The optic is repositioned at the periumbilical port, the bipolar grasper at the caudal port, the monopolar scissors at the initial optic port, and the suction device at the xiphoid process port (Fig. 9).

TIP

The assistant moves to the right side of the surgeon.

Surgical Technique

Colon Mobilization

For a *left-side nephroureterectomy*, the plane between the descending colon and the underlying Gerota's fascia is developed to allow the colon to fall medially (Fig. 10a–c).

TIP

The lateral attachments of Gerota's fascia to the abdominal wall should not be freed at this time to avoid the kidney falling medially into the operating field.

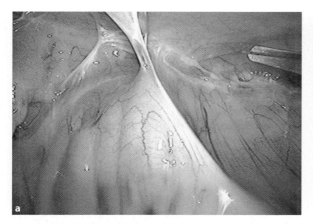

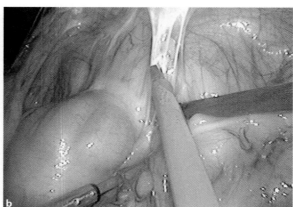

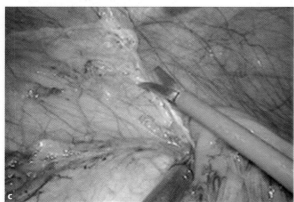

FIG. 10

a Colon attachments to abdominal wall. **b** Release of the colon attachments to abdominal wall. **c** Colon is dissected from Gerota's fascia (Gerota is not freed from abdominal wall)

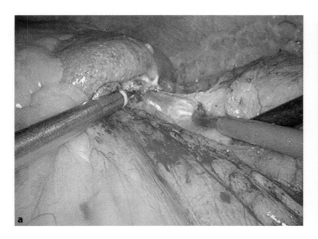

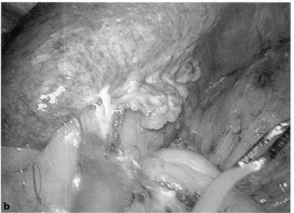

FIG. 11

a Spleen is released from kidney. **b** Spleen dissected en bloc

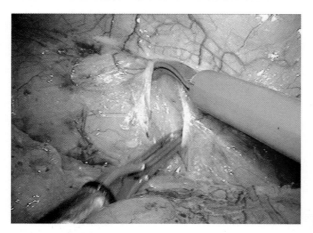

FIG. 12

Lifting of fatty tissue to expose psoas muscle

nal wall. The ascending colon is mobilized and dissected from the underlying Gerota's fascia. Colon mobilization continues caudally to the common iliac vessels.

Ureter and Gonadal Vessels Identification

Following the medial mobilization of the colon and mesocolon, the gonadal vessels are visualized. After the colon is medially retracted, the Gerota's fatty tissue at the level of the lower pole of the kidney is incised and lifted to locate the psoas muscle (Fig. 12).

> **TIP**
>
> *The correct maneuver to expose the psoas muscle is the continuous upper movement of the laparoscopic instruments to lift the fatty tissue.*

This plane of dissection is carried out cranially. The splenorenal and lienocolic ligaments are incised, allowing the spleen and the tail of the pancreas to be separated from the upper pole of the kidney. The en bloc dissection of the colon, spleen, and pancreas must be completed for adequate exposure of the renal vein (Fig. 11a,b).

For a *right-side nephroureterectomy*, the liver is cranially retracted using a grasper that is fixed to the abdomi-

The psoas is followed to expose the ureter just lateral and deep to the gonadal vessels.

By tracking the cranial course of the ureter, the plane is followed up to the renal pedicle.

The ureter and gonadal vessels are not divided at this time. Both structures are lifted and, by visualization of the psoas muscle (Fig. 13a,b) *together with the gonadal*

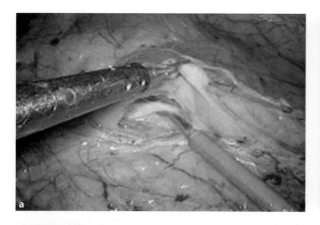

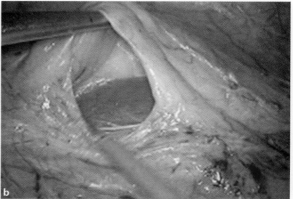

FIG. 13

a Dissection of ureter and gonadal vessels. **b** Psoas muscle

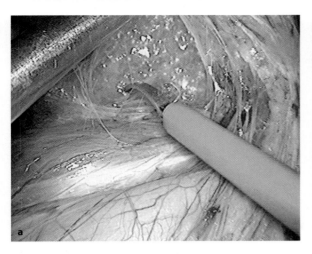
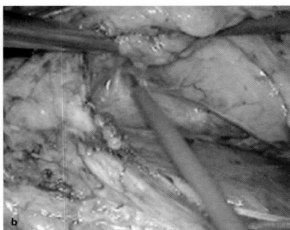

FIG. 14

a Psoas is followed cranially to hilum. **b** Ureter and gonadal vessels approaching renal hilum

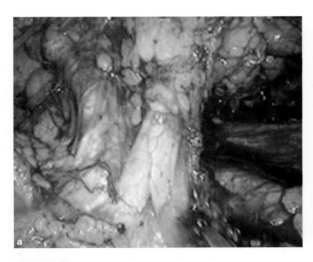
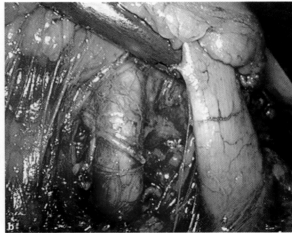

FIG. 15

a Renal hilum exposed. **b** Individual vessel dissection

vessels on the left side, followed cranially to the lower pole and hilum of the kidney (Fig. 14a,b).

The dissection of the right gonadal vein is not necessary, as it enters the vena cava on this side. Attachments between the psoas muscle and Gerota's fascia are released with sharp and blunt dissection, and small vessels to the ureter and branches of the gonadal vein are coagulated with the bipolar grasper.

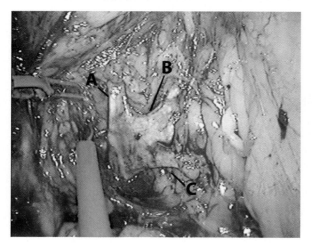

Left adrenal vein (A); Left renal vein (B); Gonadal vein (C)

Exposure and Dissection of the Renal Hilum

On the left, tracking the course of the left gonadal vein into the renal vein and firm elevation of the lower pole of the kidney on both sides assists in the identification and blunt dissection of the renal hilum. The renal vessels should be dissected separately (Fig. 15a,b).

The renal vein is dissected, taking care with the lumbar veins that drain posteriorly to the vessel. The left adrenal vein is preserved if the ipsilateral adrenal gland is not removed (Fig. 16).

> **TIP**
>
> *Dissection of the right renal vein is usually less demanding as the gonadal and lumbar veins are normally absent at this side.*

The renal artery is exposed posterior to the renal vein and dissected (Fig. 17a,b).

Renal Hilum Ligature and Transection

Hem-o-lok clips are applied to the artery.

> **TIP**
>
> *One extra-large (XL) clip secures the renal artery before the renal vein is clipped.*

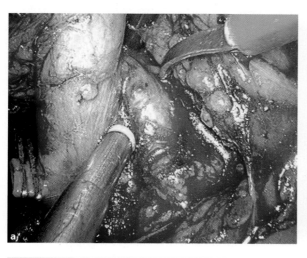
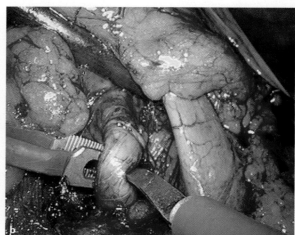

a Renal artery posterior to renal vein. **b** Dissection of the renal artery

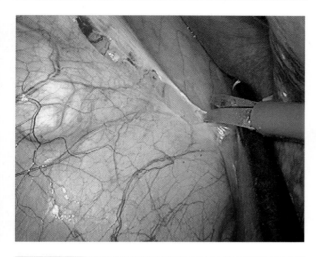

FIG. 18
Plane between kidney and liver

Three clips (XL Hem-o-lok) are used on the renal vein, which is then carefully transected.

> **TIP**
>
> *The renal vein should be flat after the renal artery clip is placed; if the vein is still filling, another renal artery should be located.*

Following division of the renal vein, clipping of the renal artery is completed (3 XL Hem-o-lok clips), and the vessel is then transected.

Mobilization of the Kidney and Adrenal Gland

Once all the hilar vessels have been divided, the dissection continues posteriorly and superiorly to the upper pole. The attachments of the kidney to the posterior and lateral abdominal wall are released by blunt and sharp dissection, taking care to coagulate the bleeding vessels. The adrenal gland can be preserved in most cases. On the right, superior retraction of the liver facilitates the dissection of the plane between the liver and the upper pole of the kidney (Fig. 18).

The ureteral dissection is continued distally as far as is technically feasible, and if an invasive ureteral lesion is suspected, the dissection should include a wide margin of surrounding tissue.

> **TIP**
>
> *The instruments are repositioned (Fig. 9)*

The ureter is double-clipped as low as possible with Ligaclip® II ML, and the remainder of the procedure can be completed through a lower ilioinguinal incision.

Kidney Extraction and Distal Ureteral Dissection

The position of the patient is maintained, and a Gibson-type incision is made. The kidney, along with the proximal and midureter, is removed, and the renal bed is inspected for bleeding. The peritoneum is incised at the level of the iliac vessels, and the incision extends medial to the medial umbilical ligament to the pelvis. The vas deferens in male patients and the round ligament in female patients is double-clipped (Ligaclip II ML) and divided. The distal ureter, now lifted and placed on traction, is dissected free between the bladder and the median umbilical ligament down to its entrance into the bladder.

> **TIP**
>
> *The bladder cuff is dissected extravesically, freeing the ureter from the surrounding detrusor muscle.*

A bladder cuff 2–3 cm surrounding the intramural ureter is delineated with the cautery, and the dissection of the intramural ureter extends into the bladder. The bladder mucosa bordering the ureteral orifice is incised, and the specimen is removed. The bladder is closed in two planes using running Vicryl 2-0 for the inner mucosal layer and interrupted Vicryl 0 for the muscular layer.

Closure of the Abdominal Wall

The abdominal wall is closed using running Vicryl 2-0 SH 1 Plus (needle ½ 21.8 mm) for the peritoneum, Vicryl 0 suture in "X" for the muscle, and running Vicryl 1 CT Plus (needle ½ 39.9 mm) for the aponeurosis. Once the abdominal wall is closed, pneumoperitoneum is reestablished, and the optic is introduced for revision of the hemostasis. A silicone Penrose drain is inserted. After evacuation of the pneumoperitoneum and removal of the trocars, the aponeurosis of the 11-mm ports is closed with a Dexon II HGU-46 suture. The skin incisions are closed with subcuticular Monocryl 3-0 C 423.

Postoperative Considerations

The nasogastric tube is removed at the end of the procedure, and the intravenous perfusion is stopped on day 1. Pain is controlled with scheduled intramuscular nonsteroidal anti-inflammatory drugs (NSAIDs) and oral analgesics. Intramuscular NSAIDs are often discontinued after 24 h. A light diet can generally be resumed on day 1 after surgery. The Foley catheter is removed on day 3 after surgery and the Penrose drain on the second postoperative day. Patients leave the hospital on the third or fourth postoperative day and can resume normal light activities, but vigorous activities and heavy lifting are limited for at least one month after surgery.

Suggested Readings

1. Rouprêt M, Hupertan V: Oncologic control after open or laparoscopic nephroureterectomy for upper urinary tract transitional cell carcinoma: a single center experience. Urology 2007 Apr; 69(4):656–661.

2. Busby JE, Matin SF: Laparoscopic radical nephroureterectomy for transitional cell carcinoma: where are we in 2007? Curr Opin Urol 2007 Mar; 17(2):83–87.

3. Rassweiler JJ, Schulze M: Laparoscopic nephroureterectomy for upper urinary tract transitional cell carcinoma: is it better than open surgery? Eur Urol 2004 Dec; 46(6):690–697.

4. Klingler HC, Lodde M: Modified laparoscopic nephroureterectomy for treatment of upper urinary tract transitional cell cancer is not associated with an increased risk of tumour recurrence. Eur Urol 2003 Oct; 44(4):442–447.

5. Gill IS, Sung GT: Laparoscopic radical nephroureterectomy for upper tract transitional cell carcinoma: the Cleveland Clinic experience. J Urol 2000 Nov; 164(5):1513–1522.

Chapter 5

Extraperitoneal Laparoscopic Radical Prostatectomy

Contents

Introduction

Initially described as "extraperitoneal endoscopic radical retropubic prostatectomy," this novel approach for the treatment of prostate cancer avoids the potential disadvantages of the transperitoneal route of dissection. As the peritoneal cavity is never entered, complications like small bowel injury, urine ascites, small bowel obstruction, and intraperitoneal bleeding without the possibility of tamponade are almost nonexistent. In addition, the occurrence of postoperative ileum is diminished. The extraperitoneal approach more closely reproduces the open retropubic radical prostatectomy technique, as the steps of the operation are almost identical. However, the pelvic and prostate anatomy is magnified during laparoscopy, making dissection of important structures much more precise. Although still considered a complex procedure, extraperitoneal laparoscopic radical prostatectomy is an evolving technique and has gained popularity in the last years. It is a safe procedure and, in experienced hands, yields oncologic and functional results equivalent to the open approach.

Preoperative Preparation

Before a patient consents to a laparoscopic radical prostatectomy, it is important to discuss the specific risks of the surgery, including the potential need to convert to the traditional open operation if difficulties arise.

The patient is admitted to the hospital one day before the surgery for bowel preparation, which includes 2 L of Colopeg® (1 envelope/L) p.o. and a Fleet® enema. Fasting starts at midnight before surgery. Thromboprophylaxis protocol is implemented with good hydra-

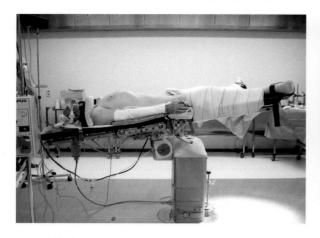

FIG. 1	FIG. 2
Patient position	Position of the legs

tion, placement of compressive elastic stockings on the lower extremities, and low-molecular-weight heparin. Enoxaparin (Clexane®, Lovenox®) 40 mg sc 1 × day or (Flaxiparine®, Fraxiparin®) 0.6 mL sc 1 × day is initiated on day 1 after the surgery and continued daily until the patient is discharged from the hospital. In selected cases, the treatment is continued for 30 days after the procedure.

> **TIP**
>
> *Thromboprophylaxis is important due to the concurrent risk factors of laparoscopy, cancer, and pelvic surgery.*

Patients also receive antibiotic prophylaxis with a single preoperative dose of intravenous second-generation cephalosporin, unless they are allergic to penicillin. Blood type and crossmatch are determined.

Patient Positioning and Initial Preparation

The surgery is performed under general anesthesia. The base of the table must be positioned below the patient's

hip to avoid elevation of the abdomen while in the Trendelenburg position (Fig. 1).

The patient is placed in the supine position with the lower limbs in abduction, allowing the laparoscopic cart to be moved closer to the surgeon and intraoperative access to the perineum (Fig. 2).

The lower buttocks must be placed at the distal end of the operating table. The upper limbs are positioned alongside the body to avoid the risk of stretch injuries to the brachial plexus and to allow for free movements of the operative team. Shoulder support is placed over the acromium clavicular joint (Fig. 3) for the Trendelenburg position.

A nasogastric tube is placed by the anesthesiologist and the stomach decompressed to avoid puncture during trocar placement and to allow additional space during extraperitoneal insufflation. The abdomen, pelvis, and genitalia are skin prepared in case conversion to an open procedure is required. An 18Fr Foley catheter with 10 mL in the balloon is introduced after the placement of the sterile drapes. The surgeon and the second assistant operate from the patient's left side, and the first assistant is placed at the opposite side of the surgeon. The laparoscopic cart is placed at the patient's feet, while the instruments table and the coagulation unit are positioned at the left side of the patient (Fig. 4).

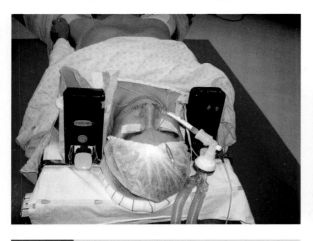

FIG. 3
Shoulder support

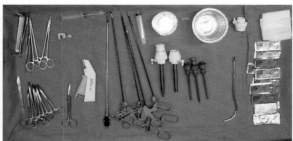

FIG. 5
Instruments table

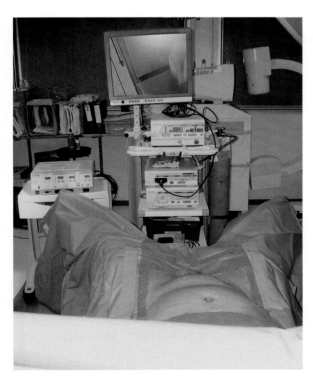

FIG. 4
Laparoscopic cart at patient's feet

Trocars and Laparoscopic Instruments

- 2 × 11 mm (optic 0° and bipolar grasper)
- 3 × 5 mm (scissors, suction device, and palpator)
- Monopolar round-tipped scissors, bipolar grasper, dissector, 5-mm suction device, needle drivers (2), and 10-mm laparoscopic optic 0° (Fig. 5)

Access and Port Placement

See Figures 6 and 7.

First Port (11 mm, optic 0°)

A cutaneous incision is made at the inferior and right margin of the umbilicus (Fig. 8).

> **TIP**
>
> *The trocar is placed in the midline to facilitate access to the right epigastric vessels in case injury to these vessels occurs during insertion of the fifth trocar.*

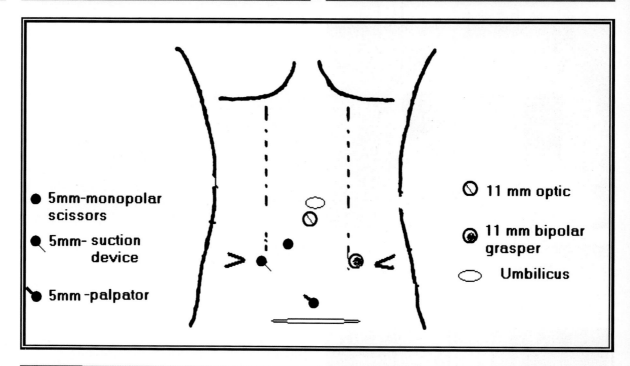

In patients with an enlarged umbilicus, where the linea alba is usually wider, the cutaneous incision should be placed more laterally, facilitating access to the right rectus abdominis muscle.

The subcutaneous fatty tissue is dissected with blunt scissors, resulting in visualization of the superficial fascia (rectus sheath). The fascia is grasped by two Kocher clamps and incised (Fig. 9a,b).

The right rectus abdominis muscle is dissected laterally, and a purse-string suture of Polysorb 0 UL 877 (needle 5/8) is placed through the superficial fascia to avoid air leakage during the procedure and to facilitate closure of the aponeurosis after the removal of the trocar.

The optic is placed inside the 11-mm trocar before insertion into the abdomen (Fig. 10). The optic and the trocar are then introduced through the skin incision at an angle of 30° (Fig. 11), following the plane above the

semicircular line of Douglas (Fig. 12) and in the direction of the prostate.

> **TIP**
>
> *The purse-string suture is "falsely" tied around the trocar by placing a Kocher clamp that blocks both threads at the level of the fascia.*

Second Port (5 mm, bladder retractor)

Following visual confirmation that the peritoneum is not opened, the insufflation line is connected, and the pressure of insufflation is switched to maximum flow. With

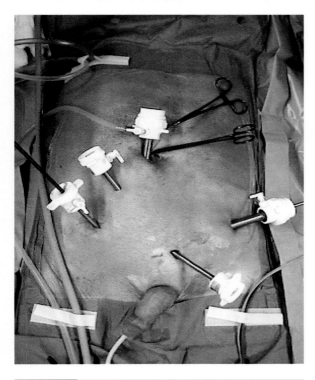

FIG. 7
Trocars in place

gentle up and down and lateral movements on the optic associated with the injected CO_2 gas, the preperitoneal space between the two epigastric vessels and the pubic arch is developed. A skin incision is made in the lower abdomen, two fingerbreadths above the pubis slightly to the left of the midline.

> **TIP**
>
> *The incision is made 50% larger than the diameter of the 5-mm trocar; it is placed slightly to the left to avoid conflict between the optic and this port.*

A 5-mm trocar is introduced (Fig. 13).

Third Port (5 mm, suction device)

The bipolar grasper is introduced through the 5-mm second port, with the tip directed toward the right anterior superior iliac spine. The Bogros space is then dissected. *The dissection should start in the angle between the epigastric vessels and the peritoneal reflection at the level of the deep inguinal ring* (Fig. 14a–c).

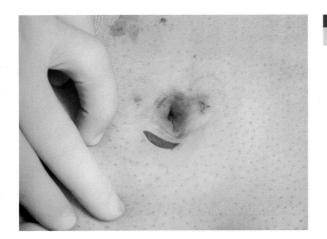

FIG. 8
Cutaneous incision to the right of midline

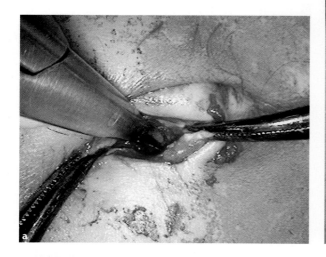

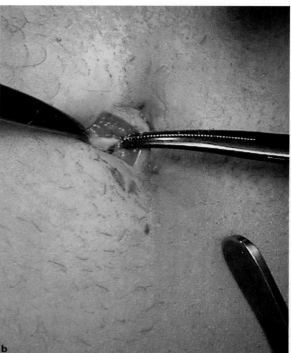

FIG. 9

a Superficial aponeurosis. **b** Aponeurosis incision

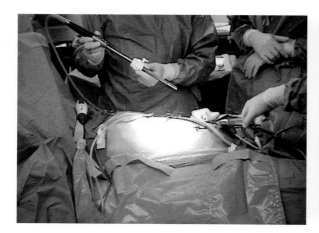

FIG. 10

Optic inside trocar

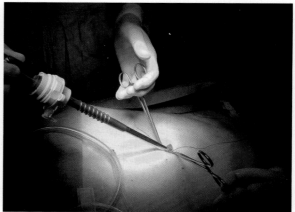

FIG. 11

Angle of trocar introduction

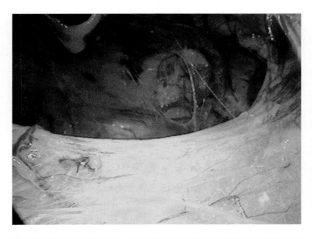

FIG. 12
Trocar follows the plane above the semicircular line of Douglas

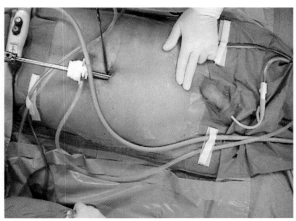

FIG. 13
Second trocar position

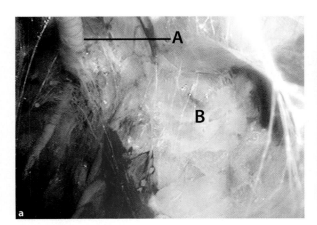

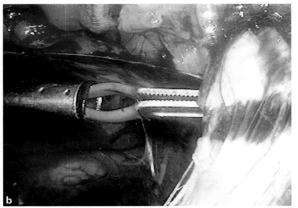

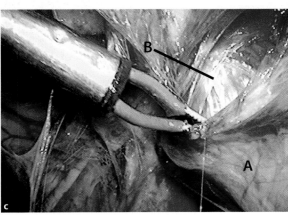

FIG. 14
Fig. 14 **a** Epigastric vessels (A); Closed Bogros space (B).
b Developing the dissection plane. **c** Peritoneal reflection
(A); Open Bogros space (B)

> **TIP**
>
> *The Bogros space is situated laterally and cranially to the Retzius space, corresponding to the retroinguinal preperitoneum. Anteriorly, it is limited by the deep layer of transversalis fascia enveloping the epigastric vessels. Medially, it is limited by the adherent zone of umbilico vesical fascia, transversalis fascia, and peritoneum, situated just behind the epigastrics. The lateral limits are the pelvic wall and the iliacus muscle. The psoas muscle corresponds to the inferior limit. The key point to visualize the Bogros space is the dissection of the epigastric vessels, which are superficial to the deep layer of transversalis fascia and in close relation to the peritoneum. If one penetrates the plane superficial to the deep layer of transversalis fascia, the bare epigastrics will be exposed, and the risk of bleeding increases by trauma to the small branching vessels—this is the wrong plane of dissection. By gently brushing the tissue away from the epigastric arcade, the right plane of dissection is usually easily visualized. The dissection follows a sagittal direction (the same direction as the fascia and the epigastrics), and the dissector gently separates the avascular plane that separates the peritoneum from the deep layer of transversalis fascia.*

The epigastric vessels are elevated by the bipolar; initially the instrument is pushed in and then pushed cranially toward the direction of the right anterior superior iliac spine. The bipolar is replaced by the optic, and the same maneuver of sagittal dissection is done to open the space for the introduction of the trocar. The grasper is then placed under the epigastric vessels. The tip is advanced laterally to the vessels, and the grasper is lifted. Holding this position, a skin incision is made from the tip of the bipolar toward the direction of the right anterior superior iliac spine, and a 5-mm trocar is placed (Fig. 15a–f).

> **TIP**
>
> *The trocar must be introduced in the same direction and inferior to the bipolar. Using this upward maneuver on the grasper, the epigastric vessels are protected from injury during trocar insertion.*

Fourth Port (11 mm, bipolar grasper)

The surgeon switches to the right side of the patient. The bipolar grasper is introduced through the right anterior superior iliac spine port, and the laparoscopic dissector is introduced through the lower abdomen port. The Bogros plane on the left side of the patient is dissected. Both instruments must be moved in the opposite up and down direction for the development of the correct plane of dissection. Then, the epigastric vessels are elevated by the dissector, and the bipolar grasper executes the same cephalad movement toward the direction of the left anterior superior iliac spine. The optic is introduced at this site and moved cranially toward the anterior left iliac spine to liberate the space for the introduction of the trocar. The grasper is then placed under the epigastric vessels. The tip is advanced laterally to the vessels, and the grasper is lifted. Holding this position, a cutaneous incision is made from the tip of the bipolar toward the direction of the left anterior superior iliac spine, and an 11-mm trocar is introduced (Fig. 16a–d).

> **TIP**
>
> *The epigastric vessels must be lifted by the bipolar, and the trocar must be placed in the same direction and inferior to the bipolar.*

> ◗ **FIG. 15**
>
> **a** Right anterior iliac crest. **b** Internal view: Epigastric vessels (A); Bogros space (B). **c** Angle of trocar introduction. **d** Trocar protruding muscle. **e** Horizontal angle of trocar introduction. **f** Trocar through the muscle

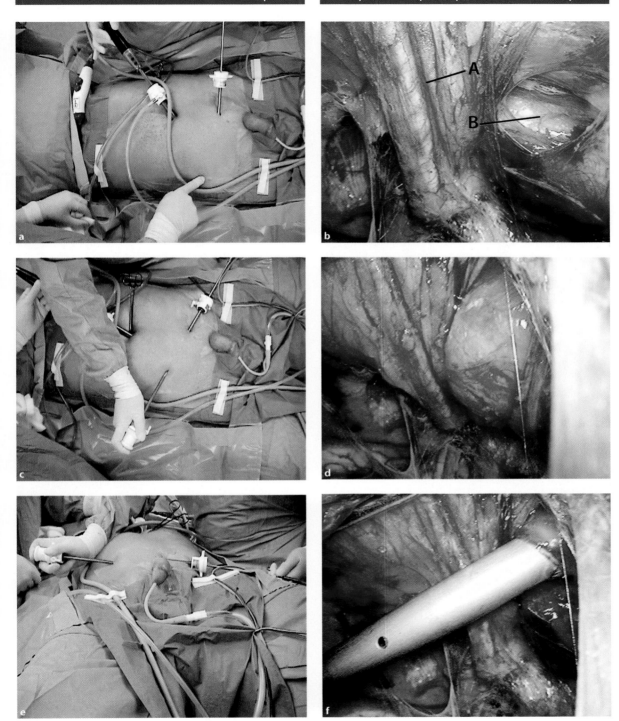

Fifth Port (5 mm, monopolar round-tipped scissors)

For the introduction of the last 5-mm trocar, a skin incision is made at a point situated at the junction of the lateral 2/3 and medial 1/3 distance between the right anterior superior iliac spine trocar and the umbilicus trocar (Fig. 17a,b).

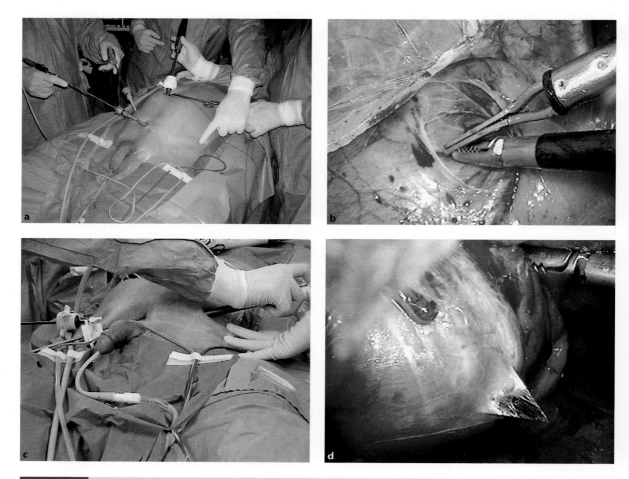

FIG. 16

a Right anterior superior iliac spine. **b** Muscle exposition. **c** Angle of trocar introduction. **d** Trocar through the muscle

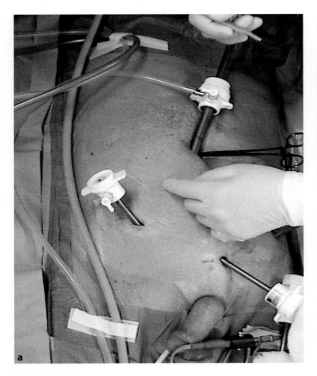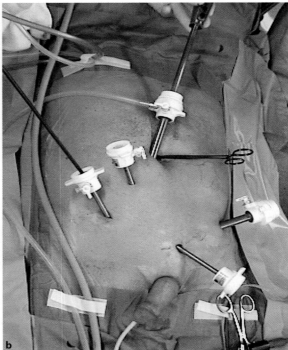

FIG. 17
a Fifth port. **b** Ports in place

The operating table is moved down and backward,
and the patient is placed in a slight Trendelenburg
position. Steps are placed for the surgeon, and the bipolar and monopolar pedals are placed over the step
(Fig. 18a,b).

Surgical Technique

Peritoneum Displacement and Exposure of the Bladder Neck

The peritoneum is cranially mobilized to increase the
extraperitoneal space. The fibroareolar and fatty tissue

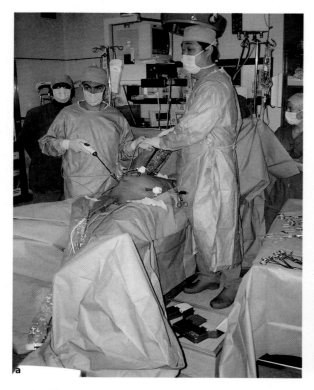

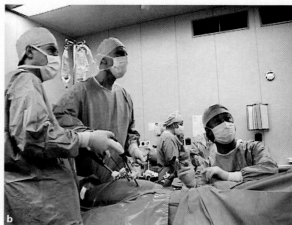

FIG. 18

a Steps under the surgeon. **b** Position of the operative team

layers between the superolateral aspect of the bladder and the medial aspect of the external iliac vein are bilaterally released. This maneuver, along with reduction of any visible pelvic wall hernia, allows for further peritoneum displacement.

> **TIP**
>
> *Every effort should be made to thoroughly coagulate the bleeding vessels during this dissection to avoid image decay throughout the procedure.*

The fatty tissue around the prostate is freed, starting laterally from the reflection of the endopelvic wall toward the midline on both sides (Fig. 19).

> **TIP**
>
> *A little traction on the tissue opens the right plane, and it is easier to start the dissection at the endopelvic fascia.*

The fibroareolar and fatty tissue attached at the level of the Santorini plexus and over the anterior surface of the prostate are pulled down toward the bladder neck with gentle but firm traction with the bipolar grasper. The superficial branch of the deep dorsal vein complex is coagulated with the bipolar grasper and cut with the cold scissors (Fig. 20).

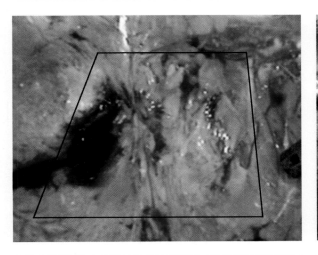

FIG. 19
Fatty tissue covering the prostate

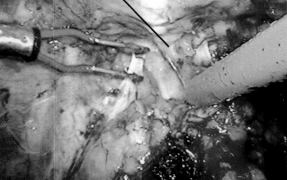

FIG. 20
Superficial veins of the Santorini plexus (A)

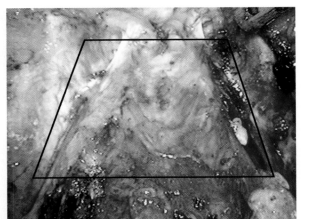

FIG. 21
Anterior prostatic surface free of fatty tissue

The fatty tissue downward traction maneuver continues until resistance is encountered, signaling the approach of the bladder neck. The dissected fatty tissue is then lifted and divided in the midline to facilitate the coagulation and transection of the vessels that overlie the bladder neck. The removal of this fatty tissue facilitates visualization and dissection of the bladder neck, which is usually located under the crossing of the fibers of the puboprostatic ligaments (Fig. 21).

> **TIP**
>
> *The superficial branch of the deep dorsal vein travels between the puboprostatic ligaments and is the centrally located vein overlying the bladder neck and prostate. It has communicating branches over the bladder itself and into the endopelvic fascia, so it is important to coagulate the vessels over the bladder neck when removing the fatty tissue at this level.*

> **TIP**
>
> *The superficial branch is transected at a safe distance from the pubic bone to prevent retraction of the vein and to permit easy vessel control in case of bleeding.*

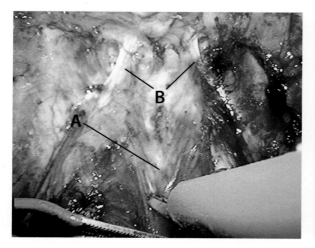

FIG. 22
Bladder neck (A) at the crossing of the fibers of the pubo-prostatic ligaments; Puboprostatic ligaments (B)

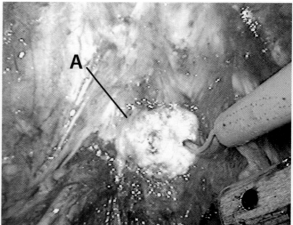

FIG. 23
Bladder neck (A) dissection

Bladder Neck Dissection and Division

The bladder neck is situated under the crossing of the fibers of the puboprostatic ligaments (Fig. 22).

A transversal incision with the monopolar scissors along with forceful counter pressure with the bipolar grasper, which is placed over the bladder, opens the superficial layer and exposes the correct plane of dissection (Fig. 23).

The incision progresses to assume an inverted U-shape to avoid dissecting through the lateral sides of the prostate. At the medial portion of the dissection, the longitudinal muscle fibers of the anterior urethral wall are exposed (Fig. 24). The urethra is dissected at its anterior and lateral aspect and then transversally transected close to the bladder neck to avoid perioperative urinary retention.

The Foley catheter is removed, and a metal 45 Fr bougie is introduced to facilitate elevation of the prostate. The dissection of the posterior plane between the bladder neck and the prostate is initiated with a U-shaped incision on the posterior urethral wall. To dissect the right lateral side of the bladder neck, the bipolar grasper with the jaws in the "closed" position is introduced into the bladder. The monopolar scissors, placed at the ex-

ternal lateral side of the bladder, touch the tip of the grasper to confirm the limits of the lateral dissection. The lateral side of the bladder is dissected, and by applying downward tension on the grasper that now holds the anterolateral bladder wall, the correct plane between the posterior bladder neck and the prostate is developed.

> **TIP**
>
> *Care must be taken not to perforate the bladder at this level as the ureteral orifices are in close proximity.*

The dissection is carried out from the lateral side to the center and continues to the other side to fully separate the bladder neck from the base of the prostate (Fig. 25).

Dissection of the Seminal Vesicles and Exposure of Denonvilliers' Fascia

The plane of longitudinal muscle fibers behind the bladder neck (Bell's muscle layer) is transversally incised to expose the vas deferens. A probe can be inserted via the

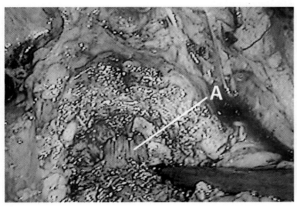

FIG. 24
Anterior urethral wall (A)

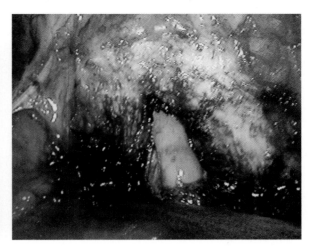

FIG. 25
Opened bladder neck with Foley catheter

suprapubic port to aid in retraction of the bladder. The vas is grasped and pulled up and laterally to expose its medial side. With a sweeping movement with the monopolar scissors, the plane between the medial side of the seminal vesicle and the Denonvilliers' fascia is released (Fig. 26).

The vas is dissected inferiorly and cut with cold scissors at its lower point.

> **TIP**
>
> *With the bipolar, coagulate the vas deferens vascular pedicle, which is situated behind the vas; after cutting this pedicle, the seminal vesicle is always exposed.*

The seminal vesicle is grasped and pulled toward the optic to facilitate exposure. The lateral pedicle of the seminal vesicle is dissected and coagulated, and following the inferior pedicle dissection and coagulation, the seminal vesicle tip is then freed. The same dissection is made on the left vas and seminal vesicle. Both structures are then grasped and lifted to facilitate dissection of the posterior plane of the prostate from the Denonvilliers' fascia. This

fascia is bluntly incised, and with downward pressure of the suction device placed at the incision, the posterior surface of the prostate is released.

There are three planes of dissection at this level (Fig. 27):

- A. A plane that extends into the prostate (the wrong plane of dissection!)

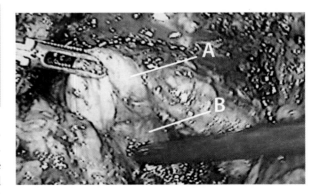

FIG. 26
Dissection of medial side of seminal vesicle (A); Denonvilliers' fascia (B)

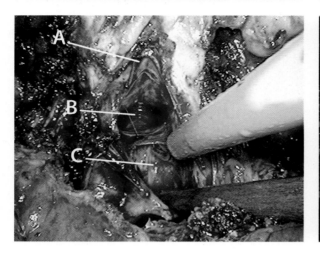

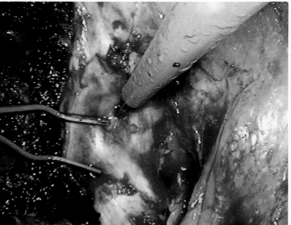

- B. A plane between the Denonvilliers' fascia and the prostate, which is the plane developed for neurovascular bundle preservation
- C. A posterior plane between the rectum and the Denonvilliers' fascia—developed in cases of wide excision of the prostate without neurovascular bundle preservation

Endopelvic Fascia and Puboprostatic Ligaments

The two layers of the endopelvic fascia are separated using gentle and forceful lateral traction and countertraction at the level of the bladder neck (Fig. 28). The fibers should not be divided close to the prostate to avoid lacerating the large veins that cross lateroposterior to the prostate. As the two layers of endopelvic fascia become more adherent moving toward the apex, they are then incised with the monopolar scissors to open the plane between the prostate and the endopelvic fascia (Fig. 29a,b).

The dissection continues upward to liberate the periurethral muscle from the prostatic apex.

> **TIP**
>
> *The muscle is bluntly separated from the lateral side of the apex with cold scissors and laterally displaced to the pelvic wall to facilitate the dorsal venous complex ligature.*

The puboprostatic ligament is cut close to the pubic bone, and the vessels are carefully dissected to expose the plane between the pubic bone and the dorsal venous complex of the penis.

> **TIP**
>
> *If bleeding occurs at this stage, the prostate is lifted with the metal bougie and pressed against the pubic bone.*

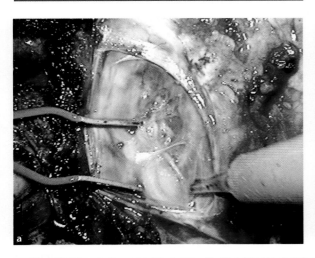
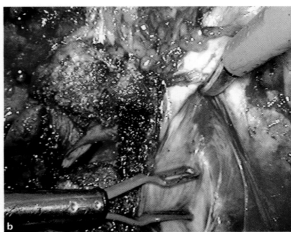

FIG. 29

a Endopelvic fascia layers divided. **b** Incision with monopolar scissors

The same dissection is done at the other side, and the dorsal venous complex is ready to be ligated (Fig. 30).

Dorsal Venous Complex of the Penis (DVC)

The dorsal vein complex at the apex of the prostate is ligated with Polysorb 0 CL 802 (needle ½ 40 mm) but not immediately cut. The needle is passed from right to left in the avascular plane between the urethra and the dorsal vein complex.

> **TIP**
>
> *The needle in the needle driver is positioned with the tip facing down to the left and with an angle of 90°.*

The needle is loaded on the tissue and elevated. Then it is advanced to the other side and finally turned to be exited at the same entrance point level on the counterlateral side (Fig. 31a,b).

> **TIP**
>
> *The common trunk of the Santorini deep venous plexus and lateral venous plexuses are covered and concealed by the prostatic and endopelvic fascia. The lateral venous plexuses course posterolaterally and communicate freely with the pudendal, obturator, and vesical plexuses. Near the puboprostatic ligaments, small branches from the lateral plexus often penetrate the pelvic sidewall musculature and communicate with the internal pudendal vein. The lateral plexus interconnects with other venous systems to form the inferior vesical vein, which empties into the internal iliac vein. With the complex of veins and plexuses anastomosing freely, any laceration of these rather friable structures can lead to considerable blood loss.*

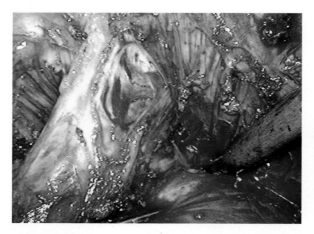

FIG. 30
Dorsal venous complex of the penis

Identification and Preservation of the Neurovascular Bundle

The neurovascular bundles are dissected and preserved, depending on anatomic and oncologic conditions. The posterolateral surface of the prostate is exposed by rolling it sideways, and sometimes the metal bougie must be removed to facilitate this maneuver. The fascial lay-

ers are incised with cold scissors, and the neurovascular bundle is gently separated from the prostate, taking care not to disrupt the prostatic capsule. The dissection is carried out in an "antegrade" or "descending" manner bilaterally, and the use of coagulation is prohibited to avoid damage to the neurovascular bundle (Fig. 32).

> **TIP**
>
> *As the neurovascular bundle usually runs at a minimal distance from the prostate at the level of the apex, the dissection of the bundle is easier at this level.*

The suction device should be positioned at a level inferior to the dissection to aspirate the blood off the operating field.

> **TIP**
>
> *The maneuver to dissect the neurovascular bundle at the right side is medial displacement of the posterolateral side of the prostate with the aid of the grasper and dissection with the monopolar scissors; for the left side, both instruments are used alternately.*

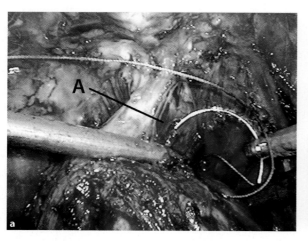

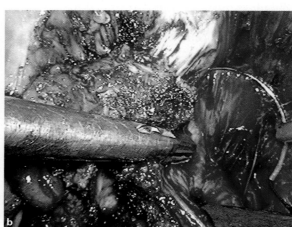

FIG. 31
a Dorsal vein complex ligation (A). **b** Angle of needle introduction (90°)

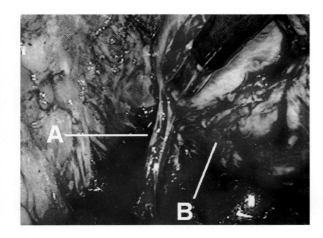

FIG. 32
Left neurovascular bundle (A); Prostate (B)

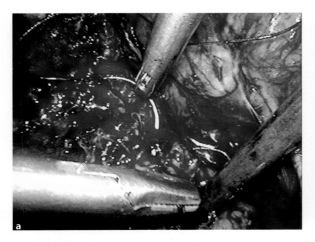

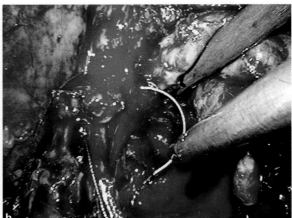

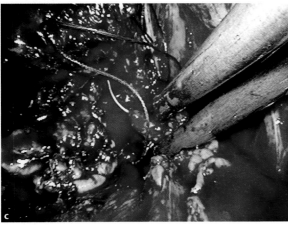

FIG. 33
a Right prostatic pedicle suturing. **b** Left prostatic pedicle suturing. **c** Prostatic pedicle – vessel ligation

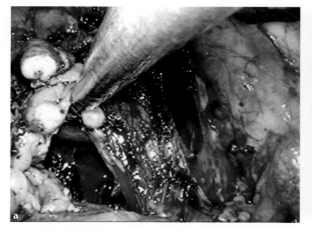

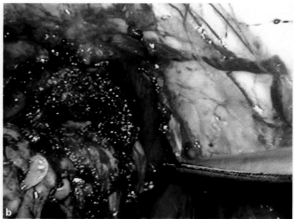

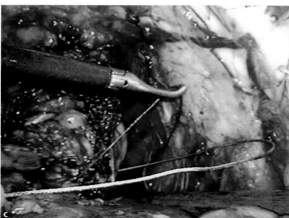

FIG. 34

a Dissector under right prostatic pedicle.
b Thread placed at the tip of the dissector.
c Threadencompasses right prostatic pedicle

The Prostatic Pedicles

There are several techniques to approach the prostatic pedicles, and they should be individualized for each patient. The prostate is lifted with the metal bougie to put the pedicles under tension. The pedicle is controlled at a safe distance from the neurovascular bundle and high on the base of the prostate. It is cut with cold monopolar scissors close to the prostate, and coagulation of bleeding vessels should be avoided at all times if potency preservation is being considered.

Technique 1

Passing a Vicryl 0 at the base of the prostatic pedicle (superficial to the neurovascular bundle), and tying the knot but not cutting the needle. The pedicle is cut with cold scissors and at the same time the pedicle vessels are carefully dissected and tied with the suture already in place. In this technique, the dissection of the neurovascular bundle begins from the posterolateral side of the prostate, and is done after the section of the vascular pedicle. (Fig. 33a–c).

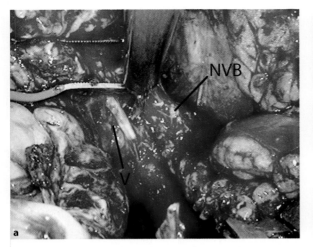

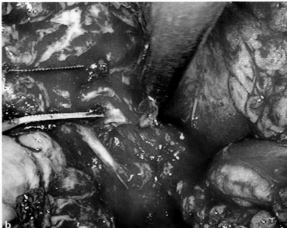

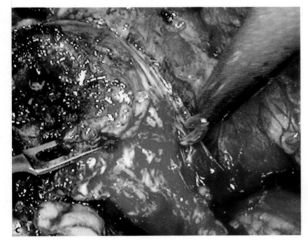

FIG. 35

a Neurovascular bundle (NVB); Prostatic pedicle vessel (V). **b** Neurovascular bundle dissected with cold scissors. **c** Neurovascular bundle displaced laterally

Technique 2

This technique involves passing a dissector underneath the pedicle close to the prostate, at right angles to its axis, and placing a simple suture of Vicryl® 0 at the tip of the clamp to be tied intracorporally. This suture should not encompass the neurovascular bundle that runs parallel to the prostatic pedicle (Fig. 34a–c). To pass the dissector through the left pedicle, the dissector is inserted through the right iliac spine port, and the suction device is placed through the paraumbilical port.

Technique 3

In the third technique, the pedicle is cut with cold scissors and, at the same time, the vessels are dissected and clipped with small size (5 mm) Hem-o-lok clips, taking care not to compromise the prostatic margins. In this technique, the dissection of the neurovascular bundle begins from the posterolateral side of the prostate and is done after the section of the vascular pedicle (Fig. 35a–c).

Technique 4

The final technique involves placing bilateral atraumatic vascular bulldog clamps (with long arms), which are introduced with the aid of a laparoscopic bulldog clamp applier. They are placed in a proximal position at the prostatic pedicle, approximately 1 cm from the prostate. After transecting the vascular pedicle, either a suture or fibrin sealant can be used to control the bleeding following removal of the vascular clamps (Fig. 36).

> **TIP**
>
> *The Denonvilliers' fascia must be longitudinally incised on both sides of the rectum for the correct placement of the long arms' bulldog clamp.*

> **TIP**
>
> *When bleeding occurs after the prostatic pedicle is transected, a running suture of Vicryl® 2-0 SH Plus is superficially placed at the internal side of the Denonvilliers' fascia, endopelvic fascia, and the vascular pedicle to control the bleeding vessel. Beginning at the internal side of Denonvilliers' fascia, the needle is passed from a cranial to a caudal direction; then at the endopelvic fascia, the needle is passed from a caudal to a cranial direction. The last suture is placed at the proximal prostatic pedicle; the needle is introduced from the lateral to the medial side, and the knot is then tied.*

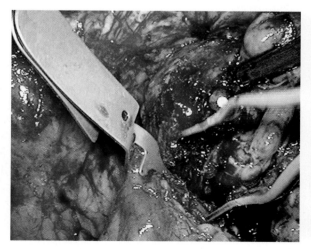

FIG. 36

Bulldog clamp at the pedicle

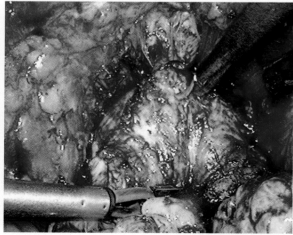

FIG. 37

Dorsal vein complex division

After the pedicles are incised, the metal bougie is pulled back from the urethra to facilitate elevation of the prostate. The posterior attachments to the Denonvilliers' fascia and the posterolateral attachments to the neurovascular bundle are released up to the apex with blunt and sharp dissection. The gland is now only connected to the deep venous complex and the urethra.

Division of the Dorsal Vein Complex and Urethra

By applying downward pressure on the metal bougie, the anterior surface of the prostate is exposed. The dorsal vein complex is divided at the apex with cold scissors, and the initial incisions are tangential to the prostate to avoid inadvertent entry into the gland (Fig. 37). By moving the metal bougie sideways, the urethra is dissected at its lateral sides until the prostatourethral junction is visualized. The metal bougie is retracted to allow the transection of the urethra as close to the apex as possible (Fig. 38).

TIP

Following the transection of the anterior wall of the urethra, the metal bougie is lifted to expose the posterior wall.

The prostate is released, and the operative site is carefully inspected for bleeding (Fig. 39). A small endobag (EndoCatch®) is introduced through the left 11-mm port, and the prostate is inserted into it. The bag with the specimen is left inside to be removed at the end of the procedure (Fig. 40).

TIP

A retractor is introduced through the 11-mm left iliac spine port, and the port is partially removed over it. The string of the bag is exteriorized through the outer surface of the port, and the port is replaced over the retractor. The bag is then pulled out and partially exteriorized, fixing the prostate away from the operative field.

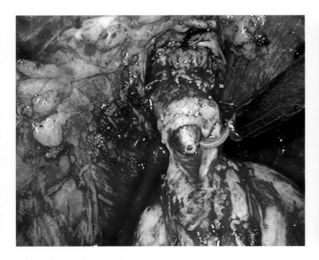

FIG. 38
Prostatourethral junction divided

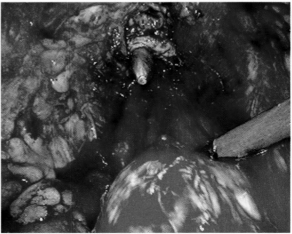

FIG. 39
Prostate released

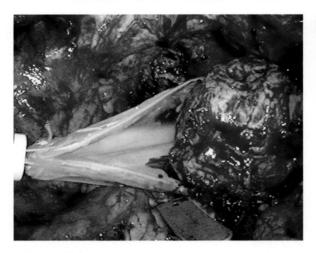

FIG. 40
Prostate inserted into endobag

Bladder Neck Reconstruction and Anastomosis

When the bladder neck needs to be reconstructed, a posterior running suture of Vicryl 2-0 is used to approximate full-thickness muscularis and mucosa, forming a tennis racket closure. It is important to visualize the position of the ureteral orifices before the closure is initiated to avoid inadvertent passage of the suture through the ureter. The bladder neck is narrowed to approximate the diameter of the urethra. The anastomosis between the bladder neck and the urethra is performed by interrupted sutures of Polysorb 2-0 GL 123 (needle ½ 26 mm). The lateral movements of the metal bougie inserted at the urethra aid in the passage of the needle. Beginning at the posterior bladder neck, a U-shaped suture is placed from the inside–outside at the bladder level; from the outside–inside of the lumen of the urethra; from the inside–outside of the lumen of the urethra; and finally from the outside–inside of the lumen of the bladder. The double-looped knot, placed inside the bladder neck, is spontaneously self-blocked due to the tension applied to the threads, allowing the bladder and urethra to be approached together (Fig. 41a–f).

> **TIP**
>
> *If tension is encountered at this step, the insufflator pressure and the Trendelenburg position are reduced to facilitate the anastomosis.*

The metal bougie is placed inside the bladder, guiding the passage of the needle for the following sutures.

Two sets of lateral sutures alternating at the 5, 7, 2, and 10 o'clock positions (Figs. 42a,b and 43) and a U-shaped suture at the 12 o'clock position with the knot on the outside are introduced (Fig. 44a–d). This U-shaped suture can also be used to close the bladder neck anteriorly, if necessary. Traction should be avoided at all times while passing the sutures to prevent tearing of the urethral wall.

> **TIP**
>
> *The right posterior sutures are done with the right hand, and the left posterior sutures are done with the left hand. For the anterior sutures, the instrument is crossed in the midline. The position of the needle on the needle holder is 2/3 posterior at a 45° angle for the posterior and anterior sutures and at a 90° angle for the lateral sutures.*

A silicone 18 Fr Foley catheter is introduced through a guide after the anastomosis is completely performed to avoid puncture of the catheter.

> **TIP**
>
> *The guide with the catheter should be laterally moved inside the bladder to confirm it is in the correct intravesical position.*

The balloon is filled with 10 mL of saline, and the integrity of the anastomosis is demonstrated by filling the bladder with 200 mL of irrigation fluid.

The prostate is removed by enlarging the left iliac spine port site.

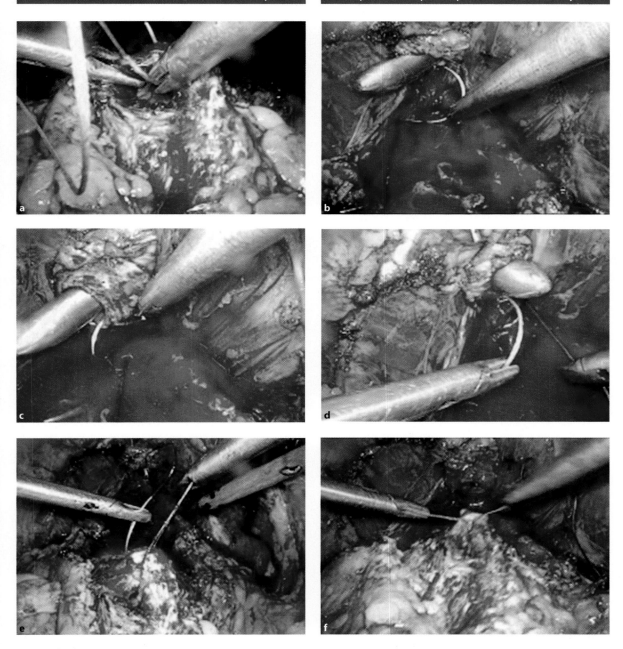

FIG. 41

Posterior vesicourethral suture sequence: **a** Initial suture at bladder neck. **b** Suture at posterior right side of urethra. **c** Suture exiting urethral lumen, right side. **d** Suture entering urethral lumen, left posterior side of urethra. **e** Final suture at bladder neck. **f** Bladder neck approaching urethra

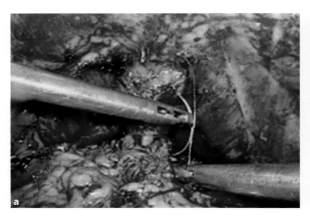 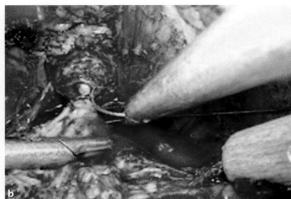

FIG. 42

Right lateral vesicourethral suture sequence: **a** Suture entering lateral bladder side. **b** Suture entering lateral urethral lumen

TIP

To enlarge the incision for the passage of the bag containing the prostate, the skin is cut at its medial end, and the fascia is cut at the lateral end to avoid injuring the epigastric vessels.

A Penrose drain is positioned close to the anastomosis and exited through the right iliac spine port site. The aponeurosis of the 11-mm port is closed with Polysorb 0 sutures, and the skin is closed with running intradermic Monocryl 3-0.

Postoperative Considerations

The nasogastric tube is removed at the end of the procedure. The patient is given appropriate analgesia as per protocol, including intravenous paracetamol during the first 24 h and major analgesics as necessary. The intravenous perfusion is stopped on day 1 after surgery, oral fluids are started the morning after surgery, and a light diet can generally be resumed on day 2. The suprapubic drain is usually removed after 48–72 h or after secretions are below 50 mL. The bladder catheter is removed on day 5 after surgery if urine is clear, but in case of persistent residual haematuria, a cystogram is performed. Normal activity is resumed four weeks after surgery.

FIG. 43

Left lateral vesicourethral suture

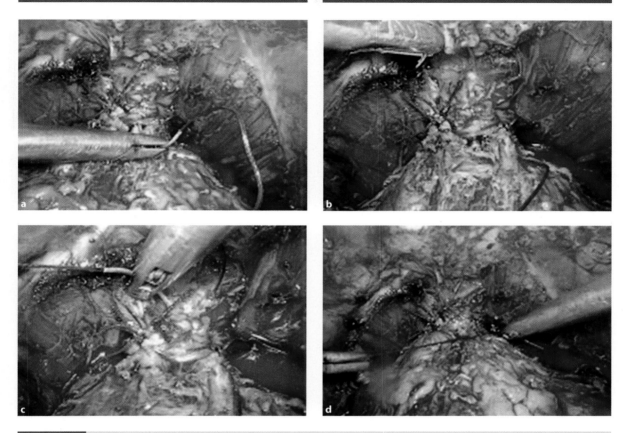

FIG. 44

Anterior vesicourethral suture sequence: **a** Initial suture at anterior bladder side. **b** Suture exiting at anterior urethral side. **c** Suture entering urethral anterior side. **d** Final knot

Suggested Readings

1. Levinson AW, Su LM: Laparoscopic radical prostatectomy: current techniques. Curr Opin Urol 2007 Mar; 17(2):98–103.

2. Stolzenburg JU, Rabenalt R: Endoscopic extraperitoneal radical prostatectomy: oncological and functional results after 700 procedures. J Urol 2005 Oct; 174(4 Pt 1):1271–1275; discussion 1275.

3. Gill IS, Ukimura O: Lateral pedicle control during laparoscopic radical prostatectomy: refined technique. Urology 2005 Jan; 65(1):23–27.

4. Erdogru T, Teber D: Comparison of transperitoneal and extraperitoneal laparoscopic radical prostatectomy using match-pair analysis. Eur Urol 2004 Sep; 46(3):312–319; discussion 320.

5. Ruiz L, Salomon L: Comparison of early oncologic results of laparoscopic radical prostatectomy by extraperitoneal versus transperitoneal approach. Eur Urol 2004 Jul; 46(1):50–54; discussion 54–56.

6. Bollens R, Vanden Bossche M: Extraperitoneal laparoscopic radical prostatectomy. Results after 50 cases. Eur Urol 2001 Jul; 40(1):65–69.

7. Raboy A, Albert P: Early experience with extraperitoneal endoscopic radical retropubic prostatectomy. Surg Endosc 1998 Oct; 12(10):1264–1267.

Chapter 6

Transperitoneal Laparoscopic Radical Prostatectomy

Contents

Introduction

Laparoscopic radical prostatectomy has become an established treatment for organ-confined prostate cancer and is increasingly performed at selected centers worldwide. The potential advantages of the transperitoneal laparoscopic radical prostatectomy compared to the extraperitoneal approach are a greater working space and reduced tension on the urethrovesical anastomosis. Furthermore, when performing extended pelvic lymphadenectomy for high-risk prostate cancer patients, the transperitoneal technique is technically less demanding than the extraperitoneal approach.

Preoperative Preparation

Before a patient consents to a laparoscopic radical prostatectomy, it is important to discuss the specific risks of the surgery, including the potential need to convert to the traditional open operation if difficulties arise.

The patient is admitted to the hospital one day before the surgery for bowel preparation, which includes 2 L of Colopeg® (1 envelope/L) p.o. and a Fleet® enema). Fasting starts at midnight before surgery. Thromboprophylaxis is implemented with good hydration, placement of compressive elastic stockings on the lower extremities, and low-molecular-weight heparin. Enoxaparin (Clexane®, Lovenox®) 40 mg sc 1 × day or nadroparin (Flaxiparine®, Fraxiparin®) 0.6 mL sc 1 × day is initiated on day 1 after the surgery and continued daily until the patient is discharged from the hospital. In selected

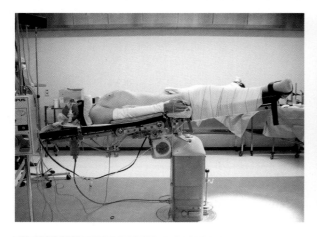

FIG. 1
Patient position

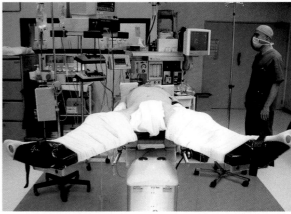

FIG. 2
Position of the legs

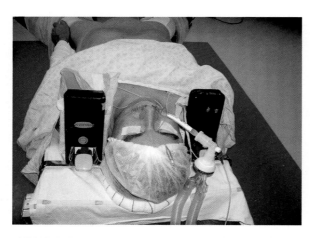

FIG. 3
Shoulder support

cases, the treatment is continued for 30 days after the procedure.

Patients also receive antibiotic prophylaxis with a single preoperative dose of intravenous second-generation cephalosporin, unless they are allergic to penicillin. Blood type and crossmatch are determined.

Patient Positioning and Initial Preparation

The surgery is performed under general anesthesia. The base of the table must be positioned below the patient's hip to avoid elevation of the abdomen while in the Trendelenburg position (Fig. 1).

The patient is placed in the supine position with the lower limbs in abduction, allowing the laparoscopic cart to be moved closer to the surgeon and intraoperative access to the perineum (Fig. 2).

The lower buttocks must be placed at the distal end of the operating table. The upper limbs are positioned alongside the body to avoid the risk of stretch injuries to the brachial plexus and to allow for free movements of the operative team. Shoulder support is placed over the acromium clavicular joint (Fig. 3) for the Trendelenburg position.

A nasogastric tube is placed by the anesthesiologist and the stomach decompressed to avoid puncture during trocar placement. The abdomen, pelvis, and genitalia are skin prepared in case conversion to an open procedure is required. An 18Fr Foley catheter with 10 mL

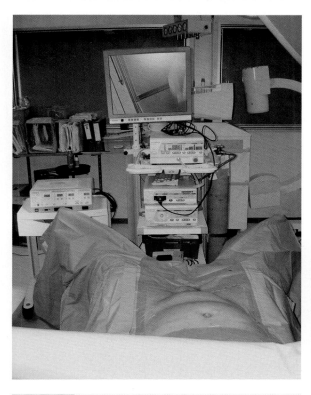

FIG. 4

Laparoscopic cart at patient's feet

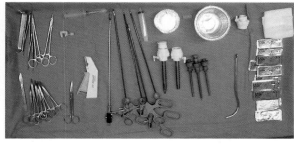

FIG. 5

Instruments table

in the balloon is introduced after the placement of the sterile drapes.

The surgeon operates from the patient's left side, and the first assistant is placed at the opposite side of the surgeon. The laparoscopic cart is placed at the patient's feet, while the instruments table and the coagulation unit are positioned at the left side of the patient (Fig. 4).

Trocars and Laparoscopic Instruments

- 2 × 11 mm (optic 0°, bipolar grasper, and 10-mm clip applier)
- 3 × 5 mm (scissors, suction device, and palpator)
- Monopolar round-tipped scissors, bipolar grasper, dissector, 5-mm suction device, 10-mm clip applier (non-disposable), needle drivers (2), and 10-mm laparoscopic optic 0° (Fig. 5)

Access and Port Placement

See Figure 6.

Veress Needle

A cutaneous incision is made at the inferior and right margin of the umbilicus.

> **TIP**
>
> *The incision should be 50% larger than the diameter of the 11-mm trocar.*

The trocar is placed in the midline to facilitate access to the right epigastric vessels in case injury to these vessels occurs during insertion of the fourth trocar. The Veress needle is introduced through the incision, and pneumoperitoneum is started (see Chap. 1, Veress Needle Introduction).

First Port (11 mm, optic 0°)

Once pneumoperitoneum is established, the needle is removed, and the 11-mm port is introduced through the same incision, perpendicularly to the abdominal wall.

> **TIP**
>
> *Pneumoperitoneum is established with an intraabdominal pressure higher than 10 mmHg.*

The optic is inserted through the port.

> **TIP**
>
> *After trocar placement and obturator removal, the trocar valve is briefly opened to check for egress of CO_2, confirming it is correctly placed inside the abdomen. The insufflator line is then connected to the trocar.*

Second Port (11 mm, bipolar grasper)

A cutaneous incision is made 2 cm medial and superior to the left anterior superior iliac spine for insertion of the 11-mm trocar.

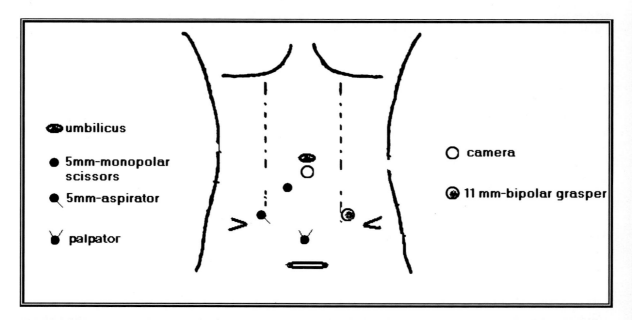

FIG. 6

Access and port placement (This figure was published in Wein: Campbell-Walsh Urology, 9th ed., Copyright Elsevier)

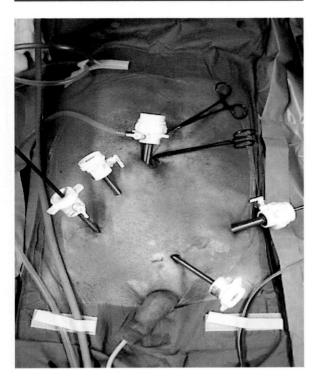

FIG. 7
Ports in place

TIP

During trocar introduction, once the cutting tip pierces the peritoneum, the position of the device is secured, allowing further gliding of the trocar to a desired site. This maneuver prevents blockage of the movements of the working instruments following an incorrect insertion.

Third Port (5 mm, suction device)

A cutaneous incision is made 2 cm medial and superior to the right anterior superior iliac spine for introduction of the 5-mm trocar.

Fourth Port (5 mm, monopolar round-tipped scissors)

For insertion of the 5-mm trocar, a cutaneous incision is made at a point situated at the junction of the lateral 2/3 and medial 1/3 distance between the right anterior iliac spine trocar and the umbilicus trocar.

TIP

Pay attention to the epigastric vessels, which can be visualized by pressing the right lateral part of the abdomen.

Fifth Port (5 mm, palpator)

A 5-mm port is medially placed two fingers above the pubis bone to complete placement of the ports (Fig. 7).

The operating table is moved down and backward, and the patient is placed in an extended Trendelenburg position. Steps are placed under the surgeon, and the bipolar and monopolar pedals are placed over the step. The surgeon, positioned higher than the assistant, can then use the working instruments (bipolar grasper and monopolar scissors) without being restrained by the assistant holding the optic in the upper midline position (Fig. 8a,b). This maneuver reduces the conflict between the operative team's arms.

Surgical Technique

Bowel Displacement

The intestine is positioned above the promontory by gently pushing back the loops of the small bowel with the aid of the Trendelenburg position. If necessary, the cecum is dissected off the posterior peritoneum to increase its mobility and assist in the cranial displacement of the small bowel. To facilitate the left-side dissection, the sigmoid and its mesocolon are laterally displaced and fixed to the abdominal wall using a monofilament 2-0 straight needle suture.

TIP

The suture needle is passed through the skin at a point lateral and cranial to the left port, placed through the appendices epiploicae of the sigmoid colon, and exited close to the entrance point. It is held in place by a Kocher clamp.

The fixation has to be released for the left pelvic wall dissection.

Pelvic Lymphadenectomy

In selected cases, a standard pelvic lymphadenectomy is bilaterally performed using a "split and roll" technique.

The posterior peritoneum above and lateral to the external iliac artery is incised with monopolar scissors. The genitofemoral nerve, which is the *lateral limit* of the node dissection, should be identified and preserved as it courses over the psoas muscle. The lymphatic tissue is lifted off the surface of the muscle and swept medially toward the iliac vessels. The tissue anterior to the iliac artery is longitudinally divided using the monopolar scissors, and the dissection extends to its lateral, medial, and inferior sides. The same dissection is done on the iliac vein.

At the *caudal limit* of the dissection, in the angle between Cooper's ligament and the inferior aspect of the external iliac vein, the nodal package over the external iliac artery and vein is clipped (XL Hem-o-lok

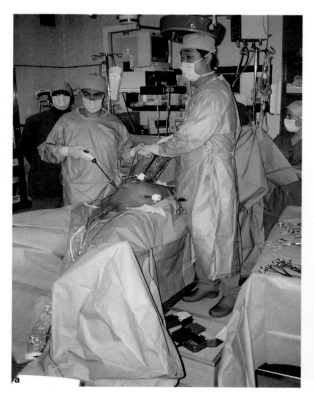

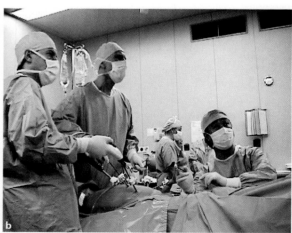

FIG. 8

a Steps under the surgeon. **b** Operative team's position

clips) and transected to reduce the occurrence of a lymphocele.

> **TIP**
>
> *The node of Cloquet is dissected at the junction of the femoral canal.*

The dissection is then carried down behind the iliac vessels, where the lateral component of the lymphatic tissue is swept under the vessels and brought to the obturator fossa. The lymphatic package is then carefully mobilized off the obturator neurovascular bundle.

> **TIP**
>
> *Care must be taken not to injure the obturator nerve.*

The dissection at this level is bordered by the obliterated umbilical artery, which is the *medial limit* of the dissection and should be preserved. Small lymphatic vessels are ligated with Ligaclip II ML. The ureter is exposed at the place where it crosses the iliac artery, and it is then medially displaced together with the medial leaf of the posterior peritoneum. The nodal dissection progresses cranially to the bifurcation of the common iliac artery, which is the *cephalad limit* of the dissection. The hypogastric artery (*posterior limit* of the dissection) is stripped of lymphatic tissue, with extreme care taken not to injure the hypogastric vein. The dissected package is then clipped (XL Hem-o-lok) and removed through the left 11-mm port.

Douglas Pouch Incision and Dissection of the Seminal Vesicles

The posterior peritoneum at the level of the Douglas pouch is transversally incised at the level of the seminal vesicles bilaterally (Fig. 9).

> **TIP**
>
> *In thin patients, the outline of the vas deferens can be followed to the seminal vesicles; otherwise, the peritoneum is incised 1–2 cm above the Douglas pouch level.*

The plane of loose areolar tissue that contains the seminal vesicles is dissected to expose its posteroinferior side (Figs. 10 and 11).

> **TIP**
>
> *Be careful not to injure the ureters that course just lateral to the seminal vesicles at this point.*

The vas deferens is bilaterally dissected, and its vascular pedicles are coagulated.

> **TIP**
>
> *Coagulate the vascular pedicle situated posterior to the vas with the bipolar forceps.*

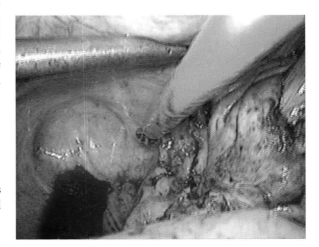

FIG. 9
Douglas pouch incision

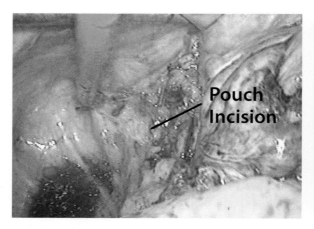

FIG. 10
Exposure of loose areolar tissue

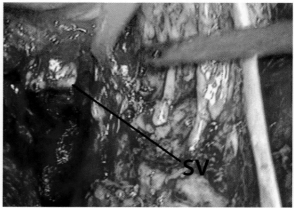

FIG. 11
Seminal vesicle (SV)

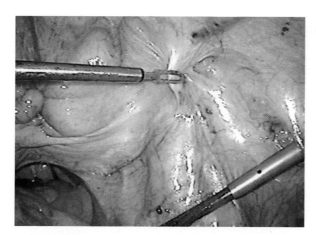

FIG. 12
Obliterated umbilical artery

> **TIP**
>
> *Denonvilliers' Fascia can be dissected at a later stage.*

Anterior Dissection—Retzius Space

The anterior peritoneum is incised medial to the obliterated umbilical artery (*medial umbilical ligament*) at the femoral ring (Fig. 12), and a plane between the prevesical fat and the lateral pelvic wall is developed.

The incision of the peritoneum continues transversally to the contralateral side, forming an arch cephalad to the bladder and inferior to the umbilicus. The urachus (*median umbilical ligament*) is identified and divided.

> **TIP**
>
> *Be careful not to injure the dome of the bladder at this level.*

Both vasa are then transected. The dissection of the seminal vesicles and its vascular pedicles, which must be thoroughly coagulated, leaves them attached only to the prostate. By lifting both vasa deferentia and the seminal vesicles with a grasper, the Denonvilliers' fascia is exposed (see Dissection of the Seminal Vesicles and Exposure of Denonvilliers' Fascia, Fig. 21).

The plane between the prevesical fat and the anterior abdominal wall is developed (Retzius space, Fig. 13),

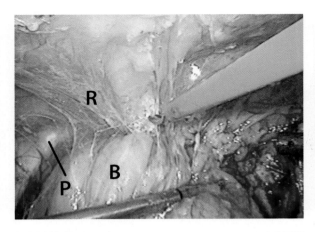

FIG. 13

Retzius space (R); Bladder (B); Pubic bone (P)

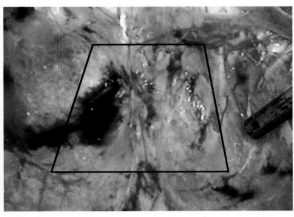

FIG. 14

Fatty tissue covering the prostate

exposing the endopelvic fascia bilaterally and the Santorini plexus medially.

> **TIP**
>
> *From this step onward, the progress of the dissection is similar to Laparoscopic Extraperitoneal Radical Prostatectomy.*

Peritoneum Displacement and Exposure of the Bladder Neck

The fatty tissue around the prostate is freed, starting laterally from the reflection of the endopelvic wall toward the midline on both sides (Fig. 14).

> **TIP**
>
> *A little traction on the tissue opens the right plane, and it is easier to start the dissection at the endopelvic fascia.*

The fibroareolar and fatty tissue attached at the level of the Santorini plexus and over the anterior surface of the prostate are pulled down toward the bladder neck with gentle but firm traction with the bipolar grasper. The superficial branch of the deep dorsal vein complex is coagulated with the bipolar grasper and cut with the cold scissors (Fig. 15).

> **TIP**
>
> *The superficial branch is transected at a safe distance from the pubic bone to prevent retraction of the vein and to permit easy vessel control in the case of bleeding.*

The fatty tissue downward traction maneuver continues until resistance is encountered, signaling the approach of the bladder neck. The dissected fatty tissue is then lifted and divided in the midline to facilitate the coagulation and transection of the vessels that overlie the bladder neck. The removal of this fatty tissue facilitates visualization and dissection of the bladder neck, which is usually located under the crossing of the fibers of the puboprostatic ligaments (Fig. 16).

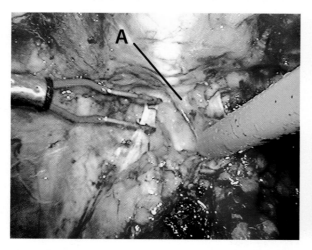

FIG. 15

Superficial veins of the Santorini plexus (A)

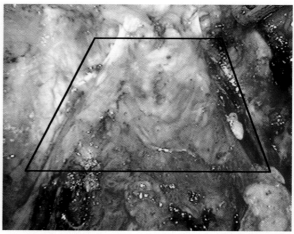

FIG. 16

Anterior prostatic surface free of fatty tissue

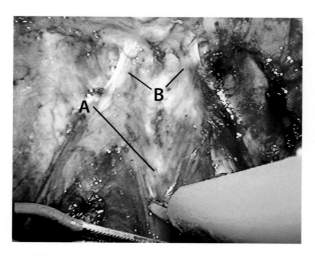

FIG. 17

Bladder neck (A); Puboprostatic ligaments (B)

TIP

The superficial veins of the Santorini plexus travel between the puboprostatic ligaments and are the centrally located veins overlying the bladder neck and prostate. There are communicating branches over the bladder itself and into the endopelvic fascia, so it is important to coagulate the vessels over the bladder neck when removing the fatty tissue at this level.

Bladder Neck Dissection and Division

The bladder neck is situated under the crossing of the fibers of the puboprostatic ligaments (Fig. 17).

A transversal incision with the monopolar scissors, along with forceful counter pressure with the bipolar grasper, which is placed over the bladder, opens the superficial layer and exposes the correct plane of dissection (Fig. 18).

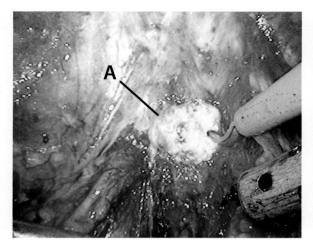

FIG. 18
Dissection of bladder neck (A)

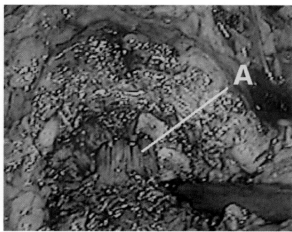

FIG. 19
Anterior wall of the urethra (A)

The incision progresses to assume an inverted U-shape to avoid entering through the lateral sides of the prostate. At the medial portion of the dissection, the longitudinal muscle fibers of the anterior wall of the urethra are exposed (Fig. 19). The urethra is dissected at its anterior and lateral aspect and then transversally incised close to the bladder neck to avoid perioperative urinary retention.

The Foley catheter is removed, and a metal 45 Fr bougie is introduced to facilitate elevation of the prostate. The dissection of the posterior plane between the bladder neck and the prostate is initiated with a U-shaped incision on the posterior urethral wall. To dissect the right lateral side of the bladder neck, the bipolar grasper with the jaws in the "closed" position is introduced into the bladder. The monopolar scissors, placed at the external lateral side of the bladder, touch the tip of the grasper to confirm the limits of the lateral dissection. The lateral side of the bladder is dissected, and by applying downward tension on the grasper that now holds the anterolateral bladder wall, the correct plane between the posterior bladder neck and the prostate is developed.

> **TIP**
>
> *Care must be taken not to perforate the bladder at this level as the ureteral orifices are in close proximity.*

The dissection is carried out from the lateral side to the center and extends to the other side to fully separate the bladder neck from the base of the prostate (Fig. 20).

Dissection of the Seminal Vesicles and Exposure of Denonvilliers' Fascia

The plane of longitudinal muscle fibers behind the bladder neck (Bell's muscle layer) is horizontally incised to expose the previously dissected retrovesical space. The vasa deferentia and the seminal vesicles are then elevated with the grasper to facilitate dissection of the posterior plane of the prostate from the Denonvilliers' fascia. If not already dissected, this fascia is bluntly incised, and with downward pressure of the suction device placed at

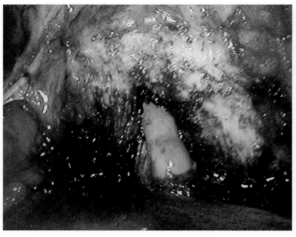

FIG. 20
Opened bladder neck with Foley catheter

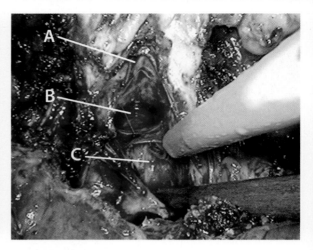

FIG. 21
Three posterior planes of prostate dissection (see text): (A), (B), and (C)

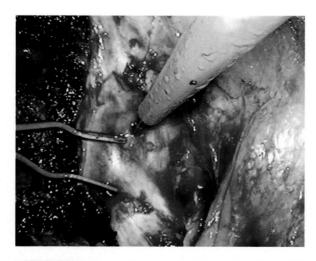

FIG. 22
Right endopelvic fascia

the incision, the posterior surface of the prostate is released.

There are three planes of dissection at this level (Fig. 21):

- A. A plane that extends into the prostate *(the wrong plane of dissection!)*
- B. A plane between the Denonvilliers' fascia and the prostate, which is the plane developed for preservation of the neurovascular bundle
- C. A posterior plane between the rectum and the Denonvilliers' fascia, developed in cases of wide excision of the prostate without neurovascular bundle preservation.

Endopelvic Fascia and Puboprostatic Ligaments

The two layers of the endopelvic fascia are separated using gentle and forceful lateral traction and countertraction at the level of the bladder neck (Fig. 22). The fibers should not be divided close to the prostate to avoid lacerating the large veins that cross lateroposterior to the prostate. As the two layers of endopelvic fascia become more adherent moving toward the apex, they are then incised with the monopolar scissors to open the plane between the prostate and the endopelvic fascia (Fig. 23a,b).

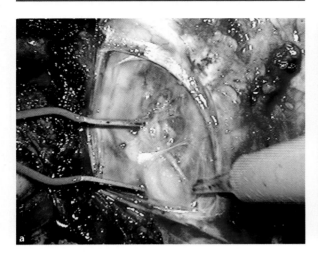
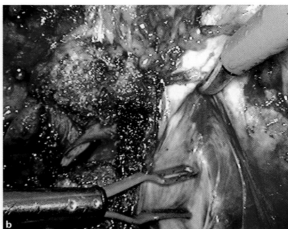

FIG. 23

a Endopelvic fascia layers divided. **b** Incision with monopolar scissors

The dissection continues upward to liberate the periurethral muscle from the prostatic apex.

> **TIP**
>
> *The muscle is bluntly separated from the lateral side of the apex with cold scissors and laterally displaced to the pelvic wall to facilitate the dorsal venous complex ligature.*

The puboprostatic ligament is cut close to the pubic bone, and the vessels are carefully dissected to expose the plane between the pubic bone and the dorsal venous complex of the penis.

> **TIP**
>
> *If bleeding occurs at this stage, the prostate is lifted with the metal bougie and pressed against the pubic bone.*

The same dissection is done at the other side, and the dorsal venous complex is ready to be ligated (Fig. 24).

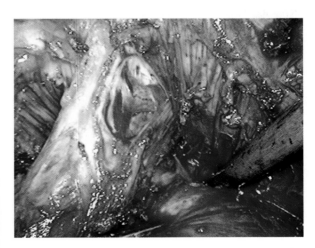

FIG. 24

Dorsal venous complex of the penis

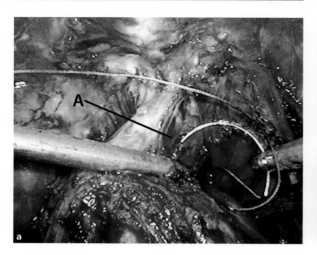
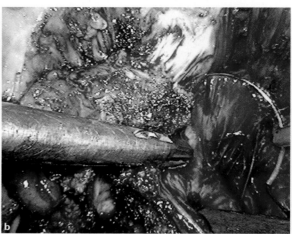

FIG. 25

a Santorini deep venous plexus ligation (A). **b** Angle of needle introduction (90°)

Dorsal Venous Complex of the Penis (DVC)

The Santorini deep venous plexus at the apex of the prostate is ligated with Polysorb 0 CL 802 (needle ½ 40 mm) but not immediately cut. The needle is passed from right to left in the avascular plane between the urethra and the dorsal vein complex.

> **TIP**
>
> *The position of the needle in the needle driver is with the tip facing down to the left and with an angle of 90°.*

The needle is loaded on the tissue and elevated. Then it is advanced to the other side and finally turned to be exited at the same entrance point level on the counterlateral side (Fig 25a,b).

Identification and Preservation of the Neurovascular Bundle

The neurovascular bundles are dissected and preserved, depending on anatomic and oncologic conditions. The posterolateral surface of the prostate is exposed by rolling it sideways, and sometimes the metal bougie must be removed to facilitate this maneuver. The fascial layers are incised with cold scissors, and the neurovascular bundle is gently separated from the prostate, taking particular care not to disrupt the prostatic capsule. The dissection is carried out in an "antegrade" or "descending" manner bilaterally, and the use of coagulation is prohibited to avoid damage to the neurovascular bundle (Fig. 26).

> **TIP**
>
> *As the neurovascular bundle usually runs at a minimal distance from the prostate at the level of the apex, the dissection of the bundle is easier at this level.*

The suction device should be positioned at a level inferior to the dissection to aspirate the blood off the operating field.

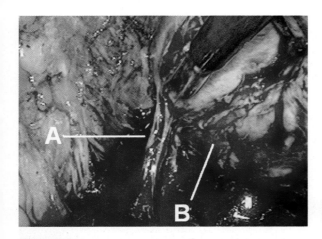

Left neurovascular bundle (A); Prostate (B)

> **TIP**
>
> *The maneuver to dissect the neurovascular bundle at the right side is medial displacement of the posterolateral side of the prostate with the aid of the grasper and dissection with the monopolar scissors; for the left side, both instruments are used alternately.*

The Prostatic Pedicles

There are several techniques to approach the prostatic pedicles, and they should be individualized for each patient. The prostate is lifted with the metal bougie to put the pedicles under tension. The pedicle is controlled at a safe distance from the neurovascular bundle and high on the base of the prostate. It is cut with cold monopolar scissors close to the prostate, and coagulation of bleeding vessels should be avoided at all times if potency preservation is being considered.

Technique 1

Passing a Vicryl 0 at the base of the prostatic pedicle (superficial to the neurovascular bundle), and tying the knot but not cutting the needle. The pedicle is cut with cold scissors and at the same time the vessels are carefully dissected and tied with the suture already in place. In this technique, the dissection of the neurovascular bundle begins from the posterolateral side of the prostate, and is done after the section of the vascular pedicle. (Fig 27a–c)

> **TIP**
>
> *Two rounds of suture should be passed at every stage, and too much space should not be left in between the running suture to avoid tearing the tissue while performing the final knot.*

Technique 2

This technique involves passing a dissector underneath the pedicle close to the prostate, at right angles to its axis, and placing a simple suture of Vicryl 0 at the tip of the clamp to be tied intracorporally. This suture should not encompass the neurovascular bundle that runs parallel to the prostatic pedicle (Fig. 28). To pass the dissector through the left pedicle, the dissector is inserted through the right iliac spine port, and the suction device is placed through the paraumbilical port.

Technique 3

In the third technique, the pedicle is cut with cold scissors and, at the same time, the vessels are dissected and clipped with small size (5 mm) Hem-o-lok clips, taking care not to compromise the prostatic margins. In this technique, the dissection of the neurovascular bundle begins from the posterolateral side of the prostate and is done after the section of the vascular pedicle (Fig. 29a–c).

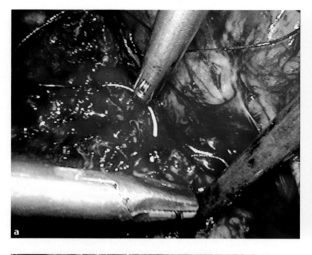

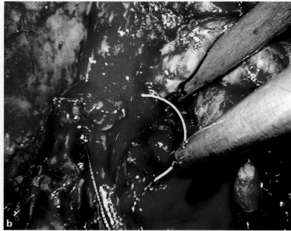

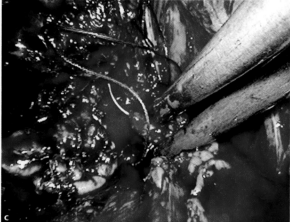

FIG. 27

a Right prostatic pedicle suturing. **b** Left prostatic pedicle suturing. **c** Prostatic pedicle – vessel ligation

Technique 4

The final technique involves placing bilateral atraumatic vascular bulldog clamps (with long arms), which are introduced with the aid of a laparoscopic bulldog clamp applier. They are placed in a proximal position at the prostatic pedicle, approximately 1 cm from the prostate. After transecting the vascular pedicle, either a suture or *fibrin sealant* can be used to control the bleeding following removal of the vascular clamps (Fig. 30).

> **TIP**
>
> *The Denonvilliers' fascia must be longitudinally incised on both sides of the rectum for the correct placement of the long arms' bulldog clamp.*

After the pedicles are incised, the metal bougie is pulled back from the urethra to facilitate elevation of the prostate. The posterior attachments to the Denonvilliers'

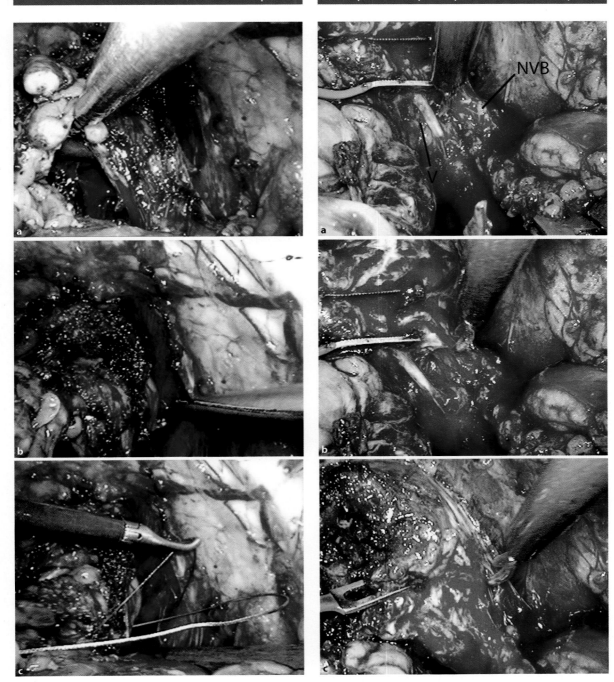

FIG. 28

a Dissector under right prostatic pedicle. b Thread placed at the tip of the dissector. c Thread encompasses right prostatic pedicle

FIG. 29

a Neurovascular bundle (NVB); Prostatic pedicle vessel (V). b Neurovascular bundle dissected with cold scissors. c Neurovascular bundle laterally displaced

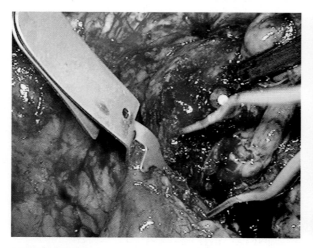

FIG. 30
Bulldog clamp at the pedicle

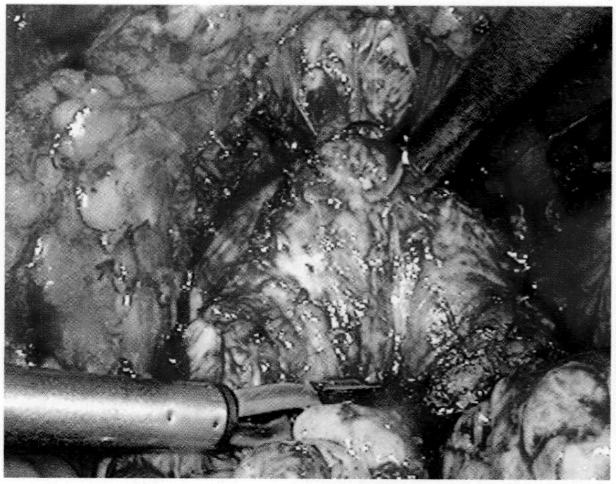

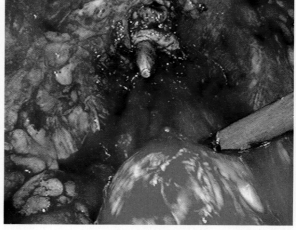

FIG. 31
Dorsal vein complex division

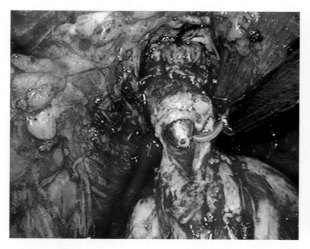

FIG. 32
Prostatourethral junction divided

FIG. 33
Prostate released

fascia and the posterolateral attachments to the neuro-vascular bundle are released up to the apex with blunt and sharp dissection. The gland is now only connected to the deep venous complex and the urethra.

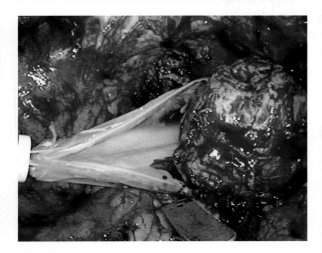

FIG. 34
Prostate inserted into endobag

The prostate is released, and the operative site is carefully inspected for bleeding (Fig. 33). A small endobag is introduced through the left 11-mm port, and the prostate is inserted into it. The bag with the specimen is left inside to be removed at the end of the procedure (Fig. 34).

> **TIP**
>
> *A retractor is introduced through the 11-mm left iliac spine port, and the port is partially removed over it. The string of the bag is exteriorized through the outer surface of the port, and the port is replaced over the retractor. The bag is then pulled out and partially exteriorized, fixing the prostate away from the operative field.*

Division of the Dorsal Vein Complex and Urethra

By applying downward pressure on the metal bougie, the anterior surface of the prostate is exposed. The dorsal vein complex is divided at the apex with cold scissors, and the initial incisions are tangential to the prostate to avoid inadvertent entry into the gland (Fig. 31). By moving the metal bougie sideways, the urethra is dissected at its lateral sides until the prostatourethral junction is visualized.

> **TIP**
>
> *It is important at this stage to follow the anatomic contours of the prostate.*

The metal bougie is retracted to allow the transection of the urethra as close to the apex as possible (Fig. 32).

> **TIP**
>
> *After cutting the anterior wall of the urethra, the metal bougie is lifted to expose the posterior urethral wall.*

Bladder Neck Reconstruction and Urethrovesical Anastomosis

When the bladder neck needs to be reconstructed, a posterior running suture of Vicryl 2-0 is used to approximate full-thickness muscularis and mucosa, forming a tennis racket closure. It is important to visualize the position of the ureteral orifices before the closure is initiated to avoid inadvertent passage of the suture through the ureter. The bladder neck is narrowed to approximate the diameter of the urethra. The anastomosis between the bladder neck and the urethra is performed by interrupted sutures of Polysorb 2-0 GL 123 (needle ½ 26 mm). The lateral movements of the metal bougie inserted at the urethra aid in the passage of the needle. Beginning at the posterior bladder neck, a U-shaped suture is placed from the inside–outside at the bladder level; from the outside–inside of the lumen of the urethra; from the inside–outside of the lumen of the urethra; and finally from the outside–inside of the lumen of the bladder. The double-looped knot, placed inside the bladder neck, is spontaneously self-blocked due to the tension applied to the threads, allowing the bladder and urethra to be approached together (Fig. 35a–f).

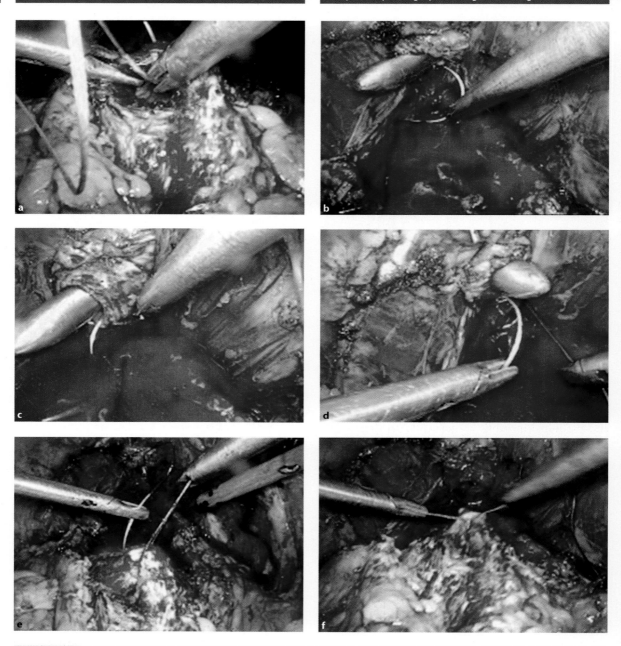

FIG. 35

Posterior vesicourethral suture sequence: **a** Initial suture at bladder neck. **b** Suture at posterior right side of urethra. **c** Suture exiting urethral lumen, right side. **d** Suture entering left posterior side of urethra. **e** Final suture at bladder neck. **f** Bladder neck approaching urethra

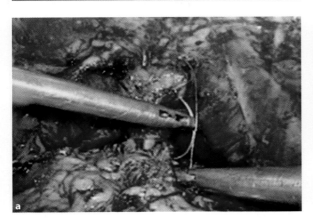 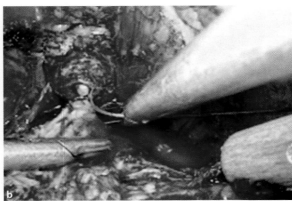

FIG. 36

Right lateral vesicourethral suture sequence: **a** Suture entering lateral bladder side. **b** Suture entering lateral side of urethra

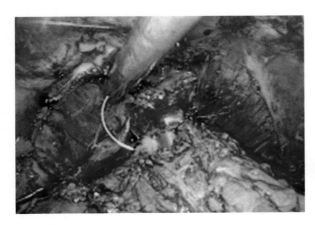

FIG. 37

Left lateral vesicourethral suture

TIP

If tension is encountered at this step, the insuf-flator pressure and the Trendelenburg position are reduced to facilitate the anastomosis.

The metal bougie is placed inside the bladder, guiding the passage of the needle for the following sutures.

Two sets of lateral sutures alternating at the 5, 7, 2, and 10 o'clock positions (Figs. 36a,b and 37) and a U-shaped suture at the 12 o'clock position with the knot on the outside are introduced (Fig. 38a–d). This U-shaped suture can also be used to close the bladder neck anteriorly, if necessary. Traction should be avoided at all times while passing the sutures to prevent tearing of the urethral wall.

TIP

The right posterior sutures are done with the right hand, and the left posterior sutures are done with the left hand. For the anterior sutures, the instrument is crossed in the midline. The position of the needle on the needle holder is 2/3 posterior at a 45° angle for the posterior and anterior sutures and at a 90° angle for the lateral sutures.

A silicone 18 Fr Foley catheter is introduced through a guide after the anastomosis is completely performed to avoid puncture of the catheter.

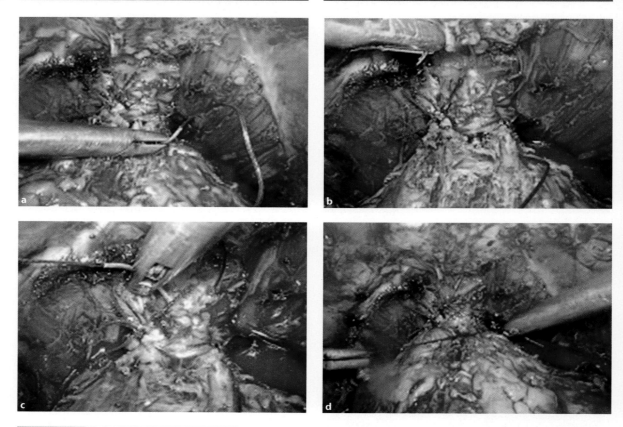

FIG. 38

Anterior vesicourethral suture sequence: **a** Initial suture at right anterior bladder side. **b** Suture exiting at right anterior urethral side. **c** Suture entering urethral left anterior side. **d** Final knot

TIP

The guide with the catheter should be laterally moved inside the bladder to confirm it is in the correct intravesical position.

TIP

To enlarge the incision for the passage of the bag containing the prostate, the skin is cut at its medial end, and the fascia is cut at the lateral end to avoid injuring the epigastric vessels.

The balloon is filled with 10 mL of saline, and the integrity of the anastomosis is demonstrated by filling the bladder with 200 mL of irrigation fluid.

The prostate is removed by enlarging the left iliac spine port site.

A Penrose drain is positioned close to the anastomosis and exited through the right iliac spine port site. The aponeurosis of the 11-mm port is closed with Polysorb 0 sutures, and the skin is closed with running intradermic Monocryl 3-0.

Postoperative Considerations

The nasogastric tube is removed at the end of the procedure. The patient is given appropriate analgesia as per protocol, including intravenous paracetamol during the first 24 h and major analgesics as necessary. The intravenous perfusion is stopped on day 1 after surgery, oral fluids are started the morning after surgery, and a light diet can generally be resumed on day 2. The suprapubic drain is usually removed after 48–72 h or after secretions are below 50 mL. The bladder catheter is removed on day 5 after surgery if the urine is clear, but in case of persistent residual haematuria, a cystogram is performed. Normal activity is resumed four weeks after surgery.

Suggested Readings

1. Levinson AW, Su LM: Laparoscopic radical prostatectomy: current techniques. Curr Opin Urol 2007 Mar; 17(2):98–103.

2. Stolzenburg JU, Schwalenberg T: Anatomical landmarks of radical prostatectomy. Eur Urol 2007 Mar; 51(3):629–639.

3. Rassweiler I, Seemann 0: Laparoscopic versus open radical prostatectomy: a comparative study at a single institution. J Urol 2003 May; 169(5):1689–1693.

4. Guillonneau B, el-Fettouh H: Laparoscopic radical prostatectomy: oncological evaluation after 1,000 cases at Montsouris Institute. J Urol 2003 Apr; 169(4):1261–1266.

5. Guillonneau B, Rozet F: Perioperative complications of laparoscopic radical prostatectomy: the Montsouris 3-year experience. J Urol 2002 Jan; 167(1):51–56.

6. Hull GW, Rabbani F: Cancer control with radical prostatectomy alone in 1,000 consecutive patients. J Urol 2002 Feb; 167(2 Pt 1):528–534.

7. Türk I, Deger S: Laparoscopic radical prostatectomy. Technical aspects and experience with 125 cases. Eur Urol 2001 Jul; 40(1):46–52; discussion 53.

8. Schuessler WW, Schulam PG: Laparoscopic radical prostatectomy: initial short-term experience. Urology 1997 Dec; 50(6):854–857.

Chapter 7

Laparoscopic Transperitoneal Radical Cystectomy

Contents

Introduction

Open radical cystectomy is the reference standard treatment for muscle-invasive bladder cancer or recurrent high-grade superficial bladder cancer. It is usually performed in elderly individuals with associated medical conditions, and the procedure can cause significant stress for patients. Following the introduction of laparoscopic radical prostatectomy and the resulting decrease in patient morbidity and recovery time, laparoscopic radical cystectomy has rapidly evolved. The oncological outcomes of the laparoscopic approach are comparable to the open procedure, and the urinary diversion can be performed completely laparoscopically or by open surgery with a minimal incision. The use of LigaSure facilitates the dissection, reducing intraoperative blood loss, operative time, and subsequent operative costs.

Preoperative Preparation

Before a patient consents to a laparoscopic radical cystectomy, it is important to discuss the specific risks of the surgery, including the potential need to convert to the traditional open operation if difficulties arise.

The bowel preparation is initiated by a non-residue diet for five days before surgery and oral self-administration of 2 L of an electrolyte solution such as Colopeg® (1 envelope/L) over two days before the procedure. The patient is admitted two days before the operation and placed on an Ensure® or Navidish® diet and bowel prophylactic antibiotics (500 mg Flagyl® + 1 g Neomicine® 3 × p.o.). Fasting starts at midnight before surgery. Thromboprophylaxis is implemented with good hydration, placement of compressive elastic stockings on the lower extremities, and low-molecular-weight heparin. Enoxaparin (Clexane®, Lovenox®) 40 mg sc 1 × day or nadroparin (Flaxiparine®, Fraxiparin®) 0.6 mL sc 1 × day is initiated on day 1 after the surgery and continued daily until the patient is discharged. In selected cases, the treatment is continued for 30 days after the procedure.

> ### TIP
>
> *Thromboprophylaxis is important due to the concurrent risk factors of laparoscopy, cancer, and pelvic surgery.*

Patients also receive antibiotic prophylaxis with intravenous second-generation cephalosporin, unless they are allergic to penicillin. Blood type and crossmatch are determined. Preoperative marking of the potential ileal conduit stoma site by a stoma therapy nurse is routine.

Patient Positioning and Initial Preparation

The surgery is performed under general anesthesia. The base of the table must be positioned below the patient's hip to avoid elevation of the abdomen while in the Trendelenburg position (Fig. 1). The patient is placed in the supine position with the lower limbs in abduction, allowing the laparoscopic cart to be moved closer to the surgeon and intraoperative access to the perineum. The lower buttocks must be placed at the distal end of the operating table. The upper limbs are positioned alongside the body to avoid the risk of stretch injuries to the brachial plexus and to allow for free movements of the operative team. A nasogastric catheter is placed by the anesthesiologist and the stomach decompressed to avoid

puncture during trocar placement. The abdomen, pelvis, and genitalia are skin prepared in case conversion to an open procedure is required. An 18Fr Foley catheter with 10 mL in the balloon is introduced after the placement of the sterile drapes.

The surgeon operates from the patient's left side, and the first assistant is placed at the opposite side of the surgeon. The laparoscopic cart is placed at the patient's feet, while the instruments table and the coagulation unit are positioned at the left side of the patient.

Trocars and Laparoscopic Instruments

- 2 × 11 mm (optic 0°, bipolar grasper)
- 2 × 5 mm (scissors, suction device, and LigaSure)
- Monopolar round-tipped scissors, bipolar grasper, 5-mm suction device, needle drivers (2), 10-mm laparoscopic optic 0°, LigaSure Atlas™ 5 mm (Tyco Healthcare)

Access and Port Placement

See Figure 2.

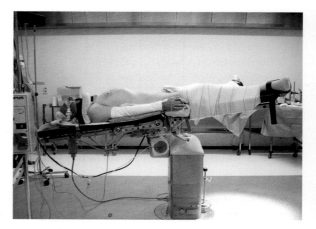

FIG. 1
Patient position

Veress Needle

A midline cutaneous incision superior to the umbilicus is made, and the Veress needle is introduced through the incision (see Chap. 1, Veress Needle Introduction).

> **TIP**
>
> *The incision should be 50% larger than the diameter of the 11-mm trocar.*

The insufflation tubing is connected to the Veress needle, the stopcock is opened, and insufflation is initiated.

> **TIP**
>
> *It is recommended to start with low flow to avoid damage to a vital structure in case the needle is malpositioned. Switch to high flow if the pressure of insufflation is increasing at a steady and normal level and there is also a tympanic percussion of the liver area.*

First Port (11 mm, optic 0°)

Once pneumoperitoneum is established, the Veress needle is removed, and the 11-mm trocar is introduced through the same incision, perpendicularly to the abdominal wall. The optic is placed through the trocar, and the insufflator line is connected to it.

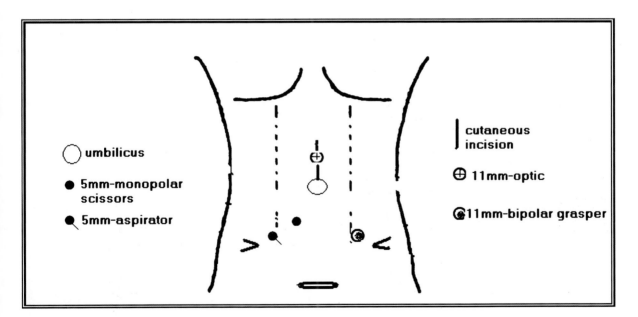

FIG. 2

Access and port placement (This figure was published in Wein: Campbell-Walsh Urology, 9th ed., Copyright Elsevier)

TIP

Care must be taken not to injure the aorta or vena cava due to the supraumbilical trocar introductio

TIP

After trocar placement and obturator removal, the trocar valve is briefly opened to check for egress of gas, confirming it is correctly placed inside the abdomen.

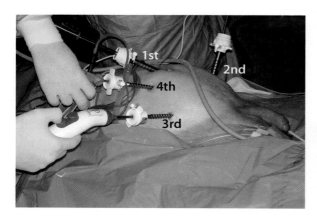

FIG. 3
Trocars in place

Second Port (11 mm, bipolar grasper)

A cutaneous incision is made 2 cm medial and superior to the left anterior superior iliac spine for introduction of the 11-mm trocar.

TIP

During trocar introduction, once the cutting tip pierces the peritoneum, the position of the device is secured, allowing further gliding of the trocar to the desired position. This maneuver prevents blockage of the movements of the working instruments following an incorrect insertion.

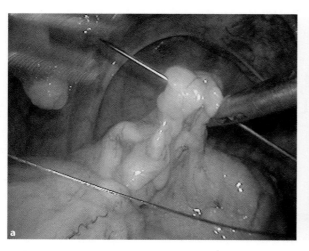

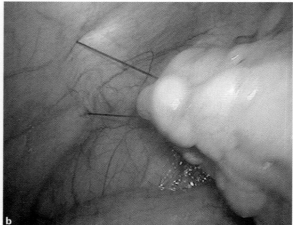

FIG. 4
a Sigmoid displacement. **b** Fixation to the abdominal wall

Third Port (5 mm, suction device)

A cutaneous incision is made 2 cm medial and superior to the right anterior superior iliac spine for introduction of the 5-mm trocar.

Fourth Port (5 mm, monopolar round-tipped scissors, LigaSure)

For insertion of the 5-mm trocar, a cutaneous incision is made at a point situated at the junction of the lateral 2/3 and medial 1/3 distance between the right anterior superior iliac spine trocar and the umbilicus trocar.

> **TIP**
>
> *The fourth trocar should be inserted at a safe distance from the potential ileal conduit stoma site.*

> **TIP**
>
> *Pay attention to the epigastric vessels, which can be visualized by pressing the right lateral part of the abdomen.*

The operating table is moved down and backward, and the patient is placed in an extended Trendelenburg position. Steps are placed under the surgeon, and the bipolar and monopolar pedals are placed over the step. The surgeon, positioned higher than the assistant, can manipulate the working instruments (bipolar grasper and monopolar scissors) without being restrained by the assistant holding the optic in the upper midline position (Fig. 3). This maneuver reduces conflict between the operative team's arms.

Radical Cystectomy in the Male

Bowel Displacement

The sigmoid is positioned above the promontory by gently pushing back the loops of the small bowel with the aid of the Trendelenburg position. If necessary, the cecum is dissected off the posterior peritoneum to increase its mobility and assist in the cranial displacement of the small bowel. To facilitate the left-side dissection, the sigmoid and its mesocolon can be laterally displaced to the left side and fixed to the abdominal wall using a monofilament 2-0 straight needle suture (Fig. 4a,b).

> **TIP**
>
> *The suture needle is passed through the skin at a point lateral and cranial to the left port, placed through the appendices epiploicae of the sigmoid colon, and exited close to the entrance point. It is held in place by a Kocher clamp.*

The fixation has to be released for the left pelvic wall dissection.

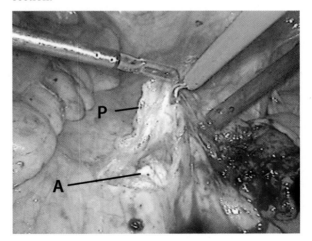

FIG. 5

Posterior peritoneal (P) incision over the common iliac artery (A)

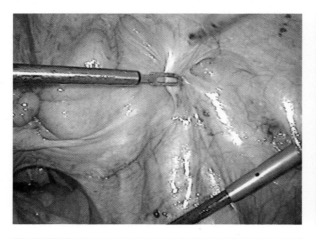

FIG. 6
Peritoneal incision extends to obliterated umbilical artery

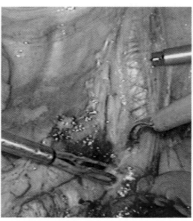

FIG. 7
Right external iliac artery exposed

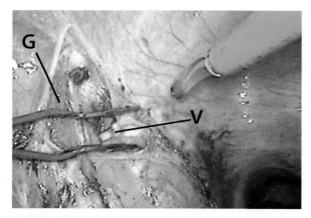

FIG. 8
Left vas (V) is coagulated and transected, and gonadal vessels (G) are laterally displaced

Retroperitoneal Incision and Exposure of Iliac Vessels

A posterior peritoneal incision is made over the right common iliac artery, and the medial peritoneal leaf is lifted to better expose the artery (Fig. 5).

> **TIP**
>
> *It is important to place traction on the peritoneum to facilitate dissection.*

The incision follows the artery caudally to a point just lateral to the medial umbilical ligament (obliterated umbilical artery), at the level of the crossing of the vas deferens (Fig. 6); cranially, the incision extends to the common iliac artery (Fig. 7).

The gonadal vessels are laterally displaced and preserved, and the vas deferens is coagulated and transected (Fig. 8).

Ureteral Exposure and Division

The ureters are identified in the retroperitoneum just cephalad to the common iliac vessels and exposed coursing over and medially at the point of bifurcation of the iliac vessels (Fig. 9). The right ureter is dissected and mobilized close to its intramural insertion into the bladder to ensure an adequate length of free ureter for reimplantation.

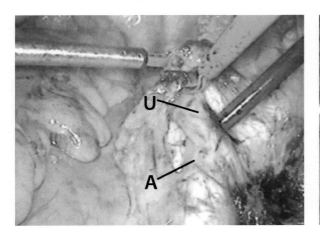

FIG. 9
Right ureter (U) crossing over the right iliac artery (A)

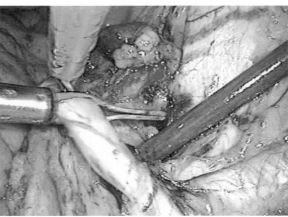

FIG. 10
Atraumatic grasping of ureter

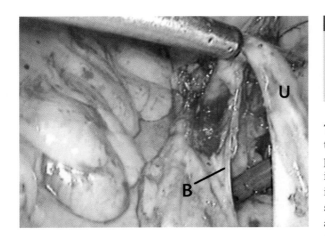

FIG. 11
Distal arterial branch (B) is coagulated; Ureter (U)

> **TIP**
>
> *A distal ureteral arterial branch from the hypogastric or inferior vesical artery can be coagulated and transected (Fig. 11).*

The ureter is double-clipped (Ligaclip® II ML) close to the bladder and transected (Fig. 12a,b). A section of the proximal ureteral segment (distal to the proximal clip) is sent for frozen-section. The proximal divided ureter is left clipped during the procedure to allow for hydrostatic ureteral dilatation, facilitating the uretero-enteric anastomosis. The ureter is then mobilized in a cephalad direction to prevent inadvertent injury, and the vascular supply derived laterally from the gonadal vessels should not be disturbed. The same dissection is done for the left ureter.

Pelvic Lymphadenectomy

The genitofemoral nerve, which is the lateral limit of the node dissection, should be identified and preserved as it courses over the right iliopsoas muscle. The right external iliac vessels are retracted medially, and the

> **TIP**
>
> *To prevent ureteral wall injury, the ureter is grasped by the atraumatic posterior part of the grasper (Fig. 10).*

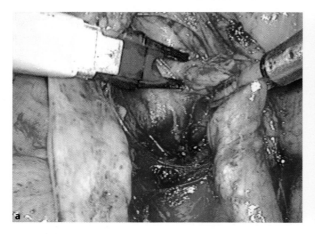

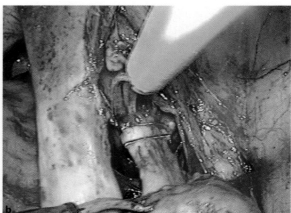

FIG. 12

a Ureteral clipping. b Ureteral transection

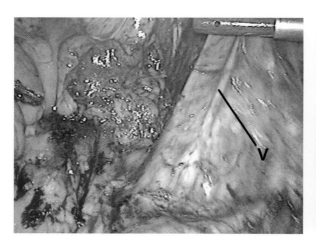

FIG. 13

"Flat" iliac vein (V)

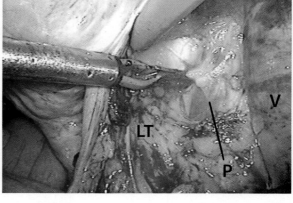

FIG. 14

Dissected tissue (LT) is swept over the psoas (P) to the obturator fossa; Iliac vein (V)

fascia overlying the muscle is incised medial to the nerve. The fibroareolar tissue is lifted off the surface of the muscle and is swept medially towards the iliac vessels.

The fibroareolar and lymphatic tissue anterior to the right external iliac artery is longitudinally divided using the monopolar scissors, and the tissue is dissected from the artery at its lateral and medial aspect.

The same dissection is performed on the right external iliac vein.

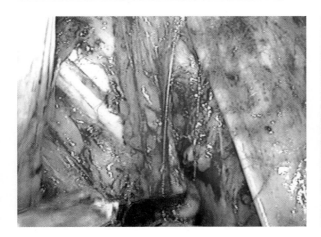

FIG. 15
Caudal limit of the dissection

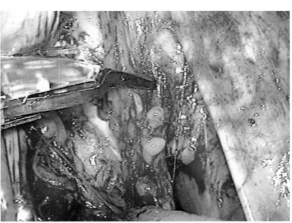

FIG. 16
Clip at nodal package

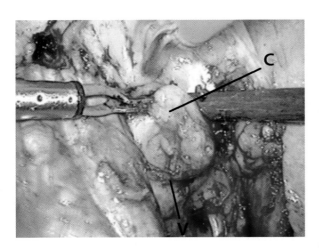

FIG. 17
Node of Cloquet (C); Accessory obturator vein (V) under the node

The dissection is then carried down behind the iliac vessels to free the lateral and medial component attached at their base. The vessels are carefully displaced laterally, and the lateral component of the fibroareolar and lymphatic tissue is swept under the vessels and along the psoas muscle and pelvic sidewall to the obturator fossa (Fig. 14).

At the *caudal limit* of the dissection, in the angle between Cooper's ligament and the inferior aspect of the external iliac vein (Fig. 15), the nodal package is double-clipped (Ligaclip II ML) and transected to reduce the occurrence of lymphocele (Fig. 16).

> **TIP**
>
> *The node of Cloquet, representing the distal limit of the dissection at this level, is dissected at the junction of the femoral canal (Fig. 17).*

> **TIP**
>
> *The external iliac vein appears flat at the standard pneumoperitoneum pressure (12 mmHg). To improve visualization, the pressure can be decreased to allow re-distention of the vessel (Fig. 13).*

A circumflex iliac vein usually runs to the external iliac vein at this location, and it can be ligated and divided if necessary.

The obturator nerve is visualized deep to the external iliac vein (Fig. 18), and the lymphatic package is then carefully mobilized off the obturator neurovascular bundle.

TIP

Care must be taken not to injure the obturator nerve (Fig. 19a,b).

The dissection at this level is bordered by the obliterated umbilical artery and lateral bladder wall, which is the *medial limit* of the dissection. Small lymphatic vessels are clipped with Ligaclip II ML.

The dissection progresses cephalad to the bifurcation of the iliac vessels, and the hypogastric artery, which is the *posterior limit* of the dissection, is visualized (Fig. 20).

TIP

For an extended lymphadenectomy, the superior limit of the dissection is initiated from the inferior mesenteric artery and extends laterally over the inferior vena cava. The fibroareolar and lymphatic tissue is dissected caudally off the aorta, vena cava. and common iliac vessels over the sacral promontory.

The lymphatic tissue is gently stripped of the hypogastric artery (Fig. 21), and care must be taken not to injure the hypogastric vein (Fig. 22).

The dissected package is then clipped (XL Hem-o-lok clips) and transected. The specimen is removed through the left 11-mm port after being placed into a bag (EndoCatch).The same dissection (Fig. 23) is done on the left side.

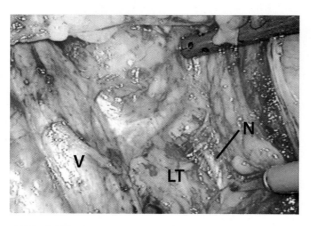

FIG. 18

Obturator nerve (N) visualized medial to the external iliac vein (V); Lymphatic tissue (LT)

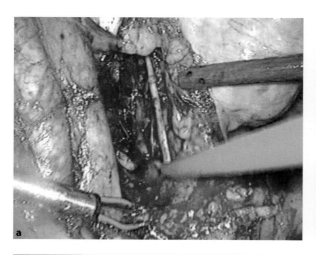

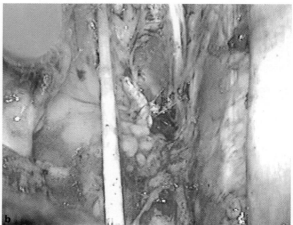

FIG. 19

a Obturator fossa. b Obturator artery and nerve

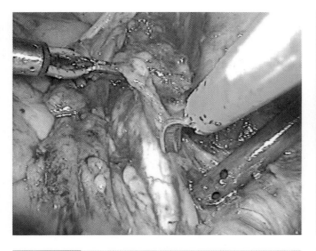

FIG. 20
Hypogastric artery

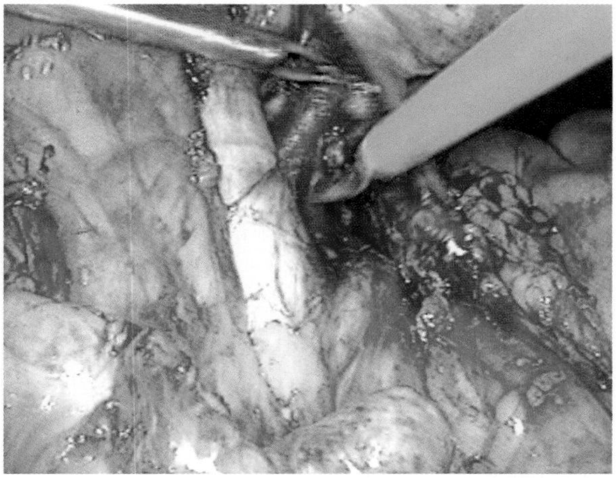

FIG. 21
Hypogastric artery dissected

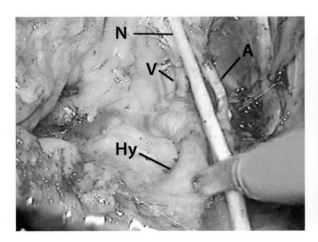

FIG. 22
Hypogastric vein (Hy); Obturator vein (V); Nerve (N); Artery (A)

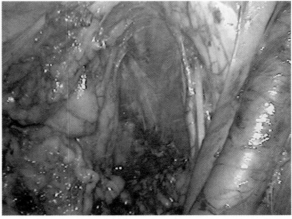

FIG. 23
Right-side dissection

Recto-Vesical Dissection

The lateral limit of the posterior peritoneum to be incised and removed with the specimen is already defined (*medial to the spermatic vessels in men and lateral to the* *infundibulopelvic ligament in women*). A transversal incision is made in the posterior peritoneum bordering the lateral aspect of the sigmoid colon (Fig. 24a,b), and the incision progresses to arrive at the level of the Douglas pouch (Fig. 25).

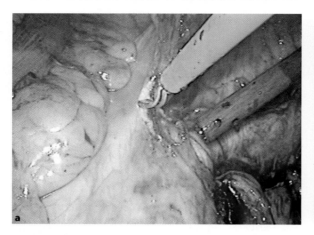

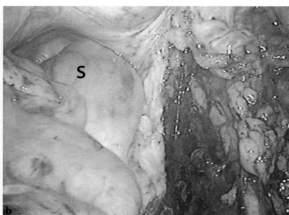

a Posterior peritoneum transversally incised. b Peritoneal incision parallel to sigmoid colon (S)

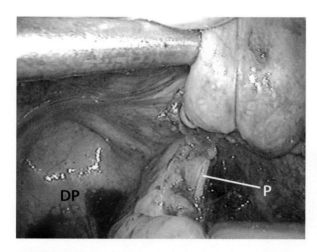

Peritoneal incision (P) extends to Douglas pouch (DP)

When started high enough, the dissection is able to leave the Denonvilliers' fascia covering the seminal vesicles. The ampullae and seminal vesicles are not dissected from the bladder and instead remain attached to it throughout the procedure (Fig. 28).

The dissection continues posterior and lateral to the seminal vesicles to expose the Denonvilliers' fascia.

TIP

To maintain potency, the dissection of this plane is done between the prostate and the Denonvilliers' fascia (above the fascia), the same as for the extraperitoneal laparoscopic radical prostatectomy with neurovascular bundle preservation. The dissection extends posterior to the prostate and to the apex.

The Douglas pouch is transversally incised close to its superior deflection, and the same procedure is made on the left side (Fig. 26a,b).

The plane of loose areolar tissue that contains the seminal vesicles is dissected to expose its posteroinferior side (Fig. 27).

The posterior layer of Denonvilliers' fascia is transversally incised to expose the perirectal fatty space. When dissecting below the fascia, the plane is followed laterally to arrive at the lateral rectal wall, creating a plane between the rectum and the levator ani muscles bilaterally.

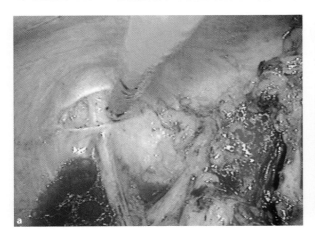
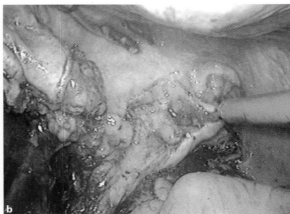

FIG. 26

a Douglas pouch transversally incised. **b** Left-side incision of posterior peritoneum

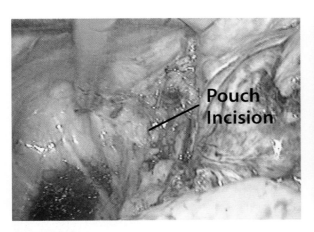
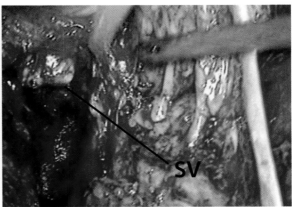

FIG. 27

Exposure of loose areolar tissue

FIG. 28

Seminal vesicle (SV)

TIP

The assistant positions the suction device at the inferior part of the dissection and pushes down on the tissue at every step of the dissection to facilitate access to the right plane.

The seminal vesicles, bladder, and prostate are then separated from the rectum, which will facilitate the second part of the bladder dissection.

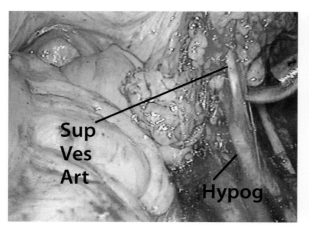

FIG. 29

Internal iliac artery (Hypog); Superior vesical artery (Sup Ves Art)

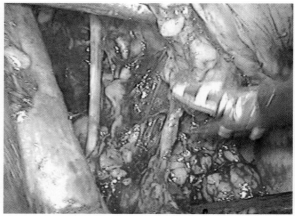

FIG. 30

LigaSure at superior vesical artery

> **TIP**
>
> *The recto-vesical dissection can be performed before the lymphadenectomy to prevent intraperitoneal contents falling into the operative field, particularly in obese patients.*

Division of the Anterior Branches of the Hypogastric Vessels—LigaSure 5mm

Following the dissection of the obturator fossa, the lateral vascular pedicle to the bladder is ready to be ligated and divided with the use of the LigaSure 5mm.

> **TIP**
>
> *The LigaSure 5 mm (settings—III and 01/01) can be used as a dissecting instrument due to its small tip.*

The hypogastric vessels are bilaterally dissected, exposing the anterior branches. The initial arterial branch is usually the superior vesical artery (Fig. 29)—the termi-

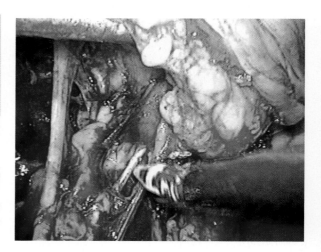

FIG. 31

LigaSure at middle vesical branches

nal section of the pervious portion of the obliterated umbilical artery—which is coagulated and transected (Fig. 30). Middle and inferior vesical arteries and branches of the middle hemorrhoidal artery that anastomose with the inferior vesical artery are also coagulated and transected (Fig. 31).

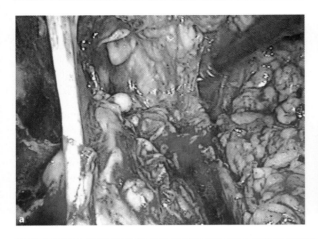
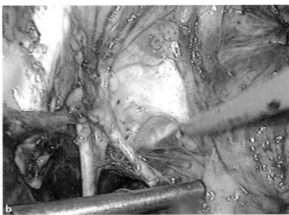

FIG. 32

a LigaSure at endopelvic fascia. **b** Endopelvic fascia opened

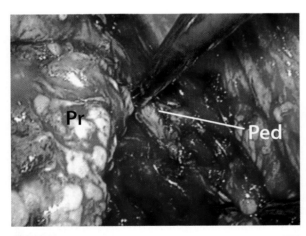

FIG. 33

LigaSure at the prostatic pedicle (Ped); Prostate (Pr)

Using the LigaSure, the posterolateral dissection of the bladder and prostate is extended caudally to the prostatic apex; laterally, the posterior pedicle is ligated and divided to the endopelvic fascia, which is opened adjacent to the prostate (Figs. 32a,b and 33).

> **TIP**
>
> *The previous dissection of the lateral border of the rectum allows for a safe dissection at this time, and opening the endopelvic fascia will help to identify the distal limit of the lateral vesical pedicle as well as aid in the control of the vessels of the prostatic apex.*

The same dissection is done on the contralateral side (Fig. 34).

Anterior Dissection of the Bladder—LigaSure 5 mm

At this point of the dissection, the bladder remains suspended through its anterior attachments. The anterior peritoneum lateral to the obliterated umbilical artery is

> **TIP**
>
> *The hypogastric artery is not ligated to avoid potential compromise of blood flow to the internal pudendal artery and possible vasculogenic impotence.*

incised from the inguinal ring to the umbilicus, and a lateral plane is developed between the prevesical fat and the pelvic wall (Fig. 35a,b).

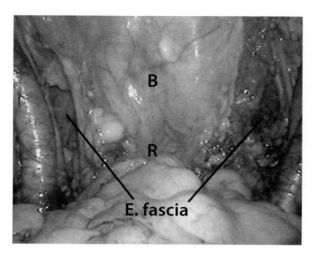

Bladder (B) pedicles bilaterally sectioned; Rectum (R); Endopelvic fascia (E.fascia) opened

The bladder can be filled with 200 mL of saline to facilitate this part of the dissection.

The inverted U-shaped incision of the peritoneum continues to the contralateral side, cephalad to the bladder and inferior to the umbilicus (Fig. 36a,b).

The urachus (median umbilical ligament) and the obliterated umbilical artery (medial umbilical ligament) are identified and divided. The bladder is emptied, and the plane between the prevesical fat and the anterior abdominal wall is further dissected (Retzius space).

The lateral portion of the pubis bone is visualized (Fig. 37a,b), and the bladder is separated from the anterior abdominal wall (Fig. 38).

With a combination of sharp and blunt dissection, the space between the lateral wall of the bladder and the pelvic side wall exposes the already opened endopelvic fascia bilaterally and the Santorini venous plexus medially. The superficial branch of the deep dorsal vein is then coagulated and divided over the anterior aspect of the prostate (Fig. 39).

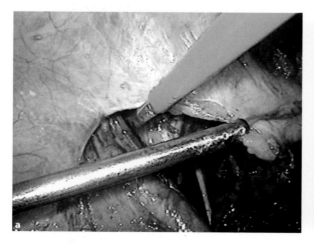
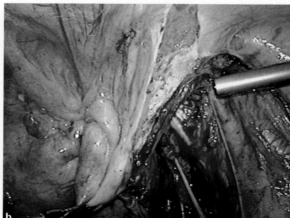

a Peritoneum lateral to the bladder incised. **b** Plane is developed between prevesical fat and pelvic wall

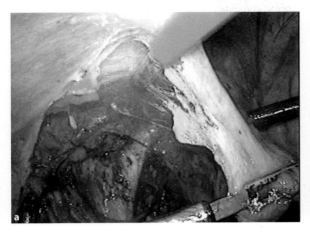
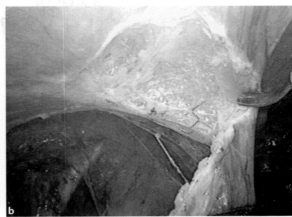

FIG. 36

a Supravesical peritoneal incision. **b** Incision extending to contralateral side

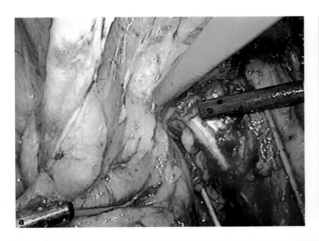
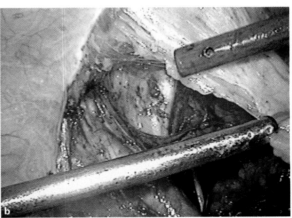

FIG. 37

a Pubic bone, right lateral portion. **b** Pubic bone, left lateral portion

The plane between the prostate and the endopelvic fascia is developed, and the neurovascular bundles are dissected and preserved, depending on anatomic and oncologic conditions.

TIP

If the patient is a candidate for nerve-sparing radical cystoprostatectomy, the steps for neurovascular bundle dissection are the same as for nerve-sparing radical prostatectomy (see Chap. 5).

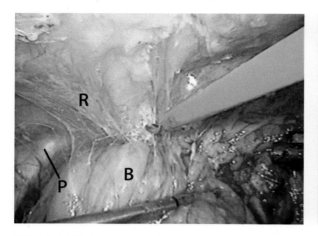

FIG. 38
Retzius space (R); Bladder (B); Pubic bone (P)

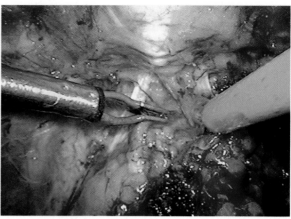

FIG. 39
Superficial branch of the deep dorsal vein

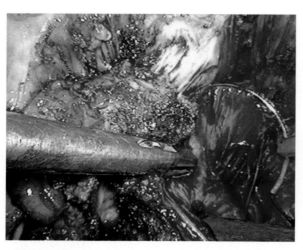

FIG. 40
Dorsal venous complex ligation

Apical Dissection

The puboprostatic ligaments are bilaterally cut, and the dorsal vein complex is ligated with Polysorb® 0 CL 802 (needle ½ 40 mm) and divided (Fig. 40).

The prostatic apex is dissected, exposing the urethra, which is ligated with Polysorb 0 CL 802 (needle

½ 40 mm) and transected following removal of the bladder catheter (Fig. 41a–c).

The proximal urinary lumen is never opened, preventing cell spillage; the distal urethra is left open. Finally, the distal insertions of Denonvilliers' fascia with rectourethral attachments are sectioned, releasing the operative specimen.

> **TIP**
>
> *Care must be taken not to injure the rectum at this level.*

The left lateral 11-mm port is removed for the introduction of a 15-mm EndoCatch® bag, and the specimen is placed inside the bag. The EndoCatch arm is removed, leaving the bag inside, and the 11-mm port is reintroduced.

A careful revision of homeostasis is performed.

The Urinary Diversion

When an ileal conduit urinary diversion is performed, an opening is made on the mesosigmoid to allow for the left ureter to be moved to the right side of the sigmoid colon. A grasper is introduced through the 5-mm port lateral to the umbilicus to hold the ureters; another grasper is introduced through the right lateral port and the distal portion of ileum that will be selected for the fashioning of the ileal conduit is secured. The optic is now placed at the left 11-mm port, and a grasper introduced through the supraumbilical 11-mm port holds and exteriorizes the EndoCatch bag string. The optic and laparoscopic instruments (except the grasper at the 5-mm port) are removed, but the abdomen is left inflated to facilitate the opening of the abdominal wall.

A small supraumbilical midline incision is made for the execution of the urinary diversion procedure in an open fashion. The specimen is removed through this incision.

A silicone Penrose drain is placed at the end of the procedure.

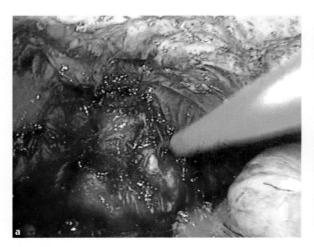
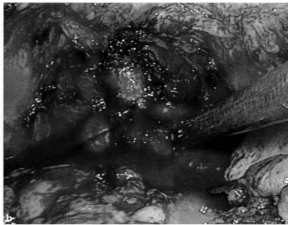
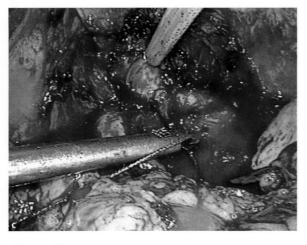

FIG. 41

a Urethral dissection. **b** Urethral ligation following catheter removal. **c** Urethral division

Radical Cystectomy in the Female

Ureteral Exposure and Division

The ureters are addressed as above.

Infundibulopelvic Ligament Division and Uterine Displacement

The right ovary is grasped and tractioned upward to better expose the infundibulopelvic ligament. The ovarian vessels in the infundibulopelvic ligament are identified, coagulated, and divided (Fig. 42a,b). The round ligament is coagulated and divided (Fig. 43). Traction can be placed on the uterus anteriorly with a Dermalon® 00 straight needle passed through the uterus.

> **TIP**
>
> *The suture needle is passed through the skin in a midline point in the lower abdomen, placed through the uterus body, exited through the skin, and loosely tied externally, allowing mobilization of the uterus if necessary.*

The same procedure is done on the left side.

Pelvic Lymphadenectomy

Pelvic lymph node dissection is bilaterally performed as described above

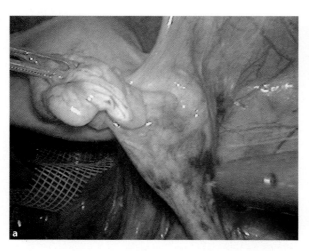

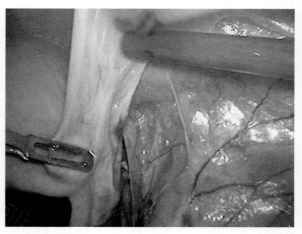

FIG. 42
a Infundibulopelvic ligament. b Coagulation of infundibulopelvic ligament

FIG. 43
Round ligament

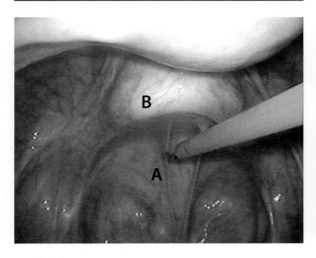

FIG. 44

Exposure of the Douglas cul-de-sac (A); Vaginal valve (B)

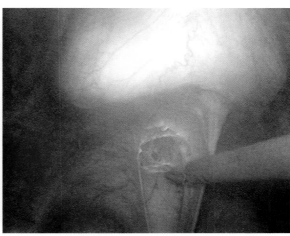

FIG. 45

Peritoneal incision at the Douglas pouch level

Recto-Vaginal Dissection

The initial steps of the dissection are the same as for the recto-vesical dissection in the male (see Recto-Vesical Dissection). When the posterior peritoneal incision approaches the Douglas pouch, a valve is introduced into

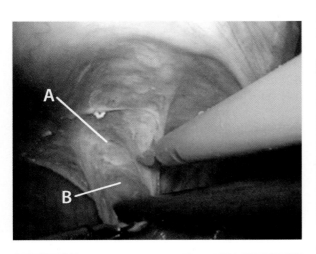

FIG. 46

a Correct plane of dissection. **b** Wrong plane of dissection

the vagina, lifting the peritoneal fold. This maneuver will aid in the exposure and facilitate the dissection of the recto-vaginal plane (Fig. 44).

The posterior peritoneum at the level of the Douglas pouch is grasped with the bipolar grasper and placed under traction. The peritoneum is incised close to its superior deflection (Fig. 45), and the inferior peritoneal lip with fatty tissue attached is pulled down to expose the correct plane of dissection (Fig. 46).

> **TIP**
>
> *Two planes of dissection are encountered at this level. The right one is between the fatty tissue and the vagina, and by applying downward traction, the avascular plane of loose areolar tissue is exposed. The wrong plane of dissection is between the fatty tissue and the rectum, and by following this plane, the chance of rectum injuries increases.*

The vaginal wall is mobilized off the rectosigmoid colon up to the level of the canal anal, and the dissection is extended laterally to the ischiorectal fossa (Fig. 47).

An incision is made at the posterior vaginal wall below the cervix.

If necessary, a small portion of the cardinal ligament can be coagulated and divided to facilitate exposure.

Division of the Anterior Branches of the Hypogastric Vessels—LigaSure 5mm

The anterior and posterior leaves of broad ligament are sharply opened and divided lateral to the uterus. The hypogastric vessels are bilaterally dissected, exposing the anterior branches. The initial arterial branch is usually the superior vesical artery, which is coagulated and transected with the use of LigaSure.

The middle and inferior vesical arteries and branches of the middle hemorrhoidal artery that anastomose with the inferior vesical artery are also coagulated and transected. The adventitious tissue surrounding the uterine vessels is dissected, and the vessels are coagulated and divided at the level of the lower uterine segment. The lateral vaginal wall is incised.

Anterior Dissection—LigaSure 5mm

Following completion of the posterior dissection, the anterior dissection is initiated and is analogous to the anterior dissection in the male cystectomy.

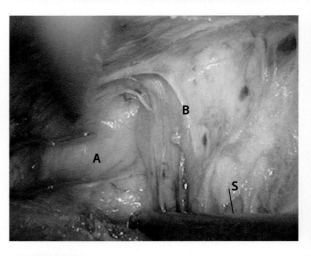

FIG. 47
Left levator ani muscle (A); Rectum (B); Suction device (S) at the inferior part of the dissection

The peritoneum cephalad to the bladder and inferior to the umbilicus is incised transversally with LigaSure, and the urachus (median umbilical ligament) and the obliterated umbilical artery (medial umbilical ligament) are identified and divided. The inverted U-shaped peritoneal incision extends along each side of the bladder, exposing the already transected round ligaments (exposed during lymphadenectomy). The bladder is emptied, and the plane between the prevesical fat and the anterior abdominal wall is developed (Retzius space), exposing the endopelvic fascia bilaterally. The endopelvic fascia is opened, allowing the dissection to be continued to the lateral aspects of the urethra. If a urethrectomy is to be performed, the pubovesical suspensory ligaments are identified and divided (these are analogous to the puboprostatic ligaments in the male). The division of the pubovesical ligaments allows the urethra and bladder to drop inferiorly. The deep dorsal vein of the clitoris is identified, ligated with Polysorb 0 CL 802 (needle ½ 40 mm) and divided. The urethra is then dissected from the dorsal vein of the clitoris, so the only remaining attachments of the specimen are the urethral meatus and a small portion of the anterior vaginal wall. The urethra is then ligated with Polysorb 0 CL 802 and divided following removal of the bladder catheter. The ovaries, fallopian tubes, uterus, and cervix are left attached by only a small portion of the anterior vagina that is now excised en bloc with the specimen.

TIP

If a continent orthotopic diversion is being considered, only the bladder neck and the initial 1 cm of urethra are removed; minimal urethral mobilization is performed distal to the urethrovesical junction. The exact location of the bladder neck is defined by in and out movements of the Foley catheter balloon, and the urethra is sharply transected at the level of the bladder neck or just distal to it. Full-thickness urethral margin biopsies are sent for frozen section.

A transvaginal approach is used if urethrectomy is to be performed. A retractor spreads the labia, and the external urethral meatus is encircled with an electrocautery knife. The entire specimen is removed transvaginally, and the vagina is laparoscopically closed with a running Vicryl 0 suture in either a posteroanterior or a vertical plane, depending on the amount of vagina left. Careful hemostasis is performed, and a silicone Penrose drain is placed at the end of the procedure.

The Urinary Diversion

The technique of urinary diversion for males is also used for the female radical cystectomy.

Postoperative Considerations

Patients are usually monitored in the intensive care unit for vital parameters and adequate pain management during the first 24 h following the procedure or until stable. Parenteral nutrition is continued until oral feeding is resumed. Early assisted ambulation is implemented. Drains stay in place until secretions drop below 50 mL and the ureteral stents (in an ileal loop diversion) are removed around day 14 after surgery. Normal activity is resumed four weeks after the procedure.

Suggested Readings

1. Haber GP, Gill IS: Laparoscopic radical cystectomy for cancer: oncological outcomes at up to 5 years. BJU Int 2007 Jul; 100(1):137–142.

2. Gerullis H, Kuemmel C: Laparoscopic cystectomy with extracorporeal-assisted urinary diversion: experience with 34 patients. Eur Urol 2007 Jan; 51(1):193–198.

3. Cathelineau X, Jaffe J: Laparoscopic radical cystectomy with urinary diversion: what is the optimal technique? Curr Opin Urol 2007 Mar; 17(2):93–97.

4. Simonato A, Gregori A: Laparoscopic radical cystoprostatectomy: our experience in a consecutive series of 10 patients with a 3 years follow-up. Eur Urol 2005 Jun; 47(6):785–790; discussion 790–792.

5. Cathelineau X, Arroyo C: Laparoscopic assisted radical cystectomy: the Montsouris experience after 84 cases. Eur Urol 2005 Jun; 47(6):780–784.

6. Moinzadeh A, Gill IS: Laparoscopic radical cystectomy in the female. J Urol 2005 Jun; 173(6):1912–1917.

Chapter 8

Laparoscopic Pelvic Lymph Node Dissection

Contents

Introduction

Prostate cancer patients with a serum PSA level of less than 10 ng/mL, a Gleason sum under 7, and a clinical stage under T2c are at low risk for pelvic nodal metastatic involvement and do not require a pelvic lymph node dissection. However, for patients with a moderate to high risk, a pelvic lymph node dissection should be performed in order to improve progression-free survival.

The anatomical lymphatic drainage of the prostate includes the obturator fossa, the external iliac, and the hypogastric artery. Laparoscopic standard lymph node dissection (obturator and internal and external iliac nodes) obtains a higher total nodal count than the modified pelvic lymph node dissection limited to the external iliac nodes or obturator fossa. It can be performed at the same time of the definitive surgery through a transperitoneal laparoscopic approach. This minimally invasive operative procedure is safe, with results and morbidity equivalent to those of open surgery.

Radical cystectomy with bilateral pelvic lymph node dissection is a standard treatment for high-grade, muscle-invasive bladder cancer. Important prognostic variables in patients with pathologic evidence of lymph node metastases are the extent of the primary bladder tumor (p stage), the number of lymph nodes removed, and the lymph node tumor burden. Although the proximal limits of the lymph node dissection remain to be better defined, selected patients with localized bladder tumor and low volume, microscopic lymph node disease can be cured with radical cystectomy and lymphadenectomy.

Preoperative Preparation

This procedure is usually performed at the time of transperitoneal laparoscopic radical prostatectomy or transperitoneal laparoscopic cystectomy. Before a patient consents to the procedures, it is important to discuss the specific risks of the surgery, including the potential need to convert to the traditional open operation if difficulties arise.

The patient is admitted to the hospital the night before the surgery for bowel preparation as for laparoscopic radical prostatectomy (see Chap. 6) or laparoscopic radical cystectomy (see Chap. 7). Fasting starts at midnight before surgery. Thromboprophylaxis is implemented with good hydration, placement of compressive elastic stockings on the lower extremities, and low-molecular-weight heparin. Enoxaparin (Clexane®, Lovenox®) 40 mg sc 1 × day or nadroparin (Flaxiparine®, Fraxiparin®) 0.6 mL sc 1 × day is initiated on day 1 after the surgery and continued daily until the patient is discharged from the hospital. In selected cases, the treatment is continued for 30 days after the procedure.

> **TIP**
>
> *Thromboprophylaxis is important due to the concurrent risk factors of laparoscopy, cancer, and pelvic surgery.*

Patients also receive antibiotic prophylaxis with a single preoperative dose of intravenous second-generation cephalosporin, unless they are allergic to penicillin. Blood type and crossmatch are determined.

Patient Positioning and Initial Preparation

The surgery is performed under general anesthesia. The base of the table must be positioned below the patient's hip to avoid elevation of the abdomen while in the Trendelenburg position. The patient is placed in the supine position with the lower limbs in abduction, allowing the laparoscopic cart to be moved closer to the surgeon and intraoperative access to the perineum. The lower buttocks must be placed at the distal end of the operating table. The upper limbs are positioned alongside the body to avoid the risk of stretch injuries to the brachial plexus and to allow for free movements of the operative team. A nasogastric catheter is placed by the anesthesiologist and the stomach decompressed to avoid puncture during trocar placement. The abdomen, pelvis, and genitalia are skin prepared in case conversion to an open procedure is required. An 18Fr Foley catheter with 10 mL in the balloon is introduced after the placement of the sterile drapes.

The surgeon operates from the patient's left side, and the first assistant is placed at the opposite side of the surgeon. The laparoscopic cart is placed at the patient's feet, while the instruments table and the coagulation unit are positioned at the left side of the patient.

Trocars and Laparoscopic Instruments

- 2 × 11 mm (optic 0° and bipolar grasper)
- 2 × 5 mm (scissors and suction device)

> **TIP**
>
> *3 × 5 mm for transperitoneal laparoscopic radical prostatectomy*

- Monopolar round-tipped scissors, bipolar grasper, 5-mm suction device, needle drivers (2), and 10-mm laparoscopic optic 0°

Access and Port Placement

See Figures 1 and 2.

Veress Needle

A midline cutaneous incision superior to the umbilicus is made for bladder cancer lymphadenectomy and at the inferior and right margin of the umbilicus for prostate cancer lymphadenectomy.

The Veress needle is introduced through the incision (see Chap. 1, Veress Needle Introduction).

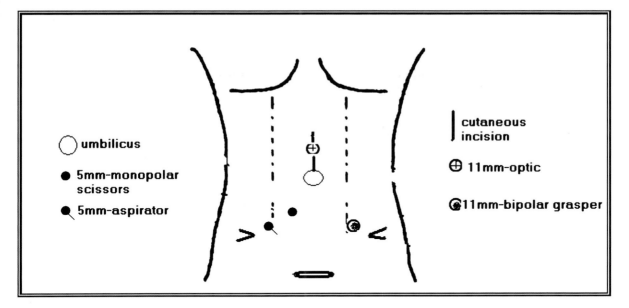

FIG. 1

Lymph node dissection for bladder cancer (This figure was published in Wein: Campbell-Walsh Urology, 9th ed., Copyright Elsevier)

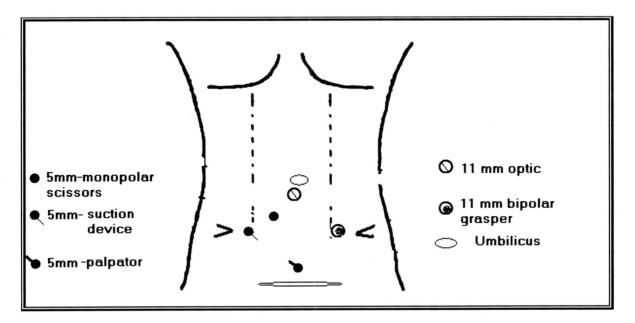

FIG. 2

Lymph node dissection for prostate cancer (This figure was published in Wein: Campbell-Walsh Urology, 9th ed., Copyright Elsevier)

The insufflation line is connected to the Veress needle, the stopcock is opened, and insufflation is initiated.

> **TIP**
>
> *It is recommended to start with low flow to avoid damage to a vital structure in case the needle is malpositioned. Switch to high flow if the pressure of insufflation is increasing at a steady and normal level and there is also a tympanic percussion of the liver area.*

First Port (11 mm, optic 0°)

Once pneumoperitoneum is established, the Veress needle is removed, and the 11-mm trocar is introduced through the same incision, perpendicularly to the abdominal wall. The optic is placed through the trocar, and the insufflation tubing is connected to it.

Second Port (11 mm, bipolar grasper)

A cutaneous incision is made 2 cm medial and superior to the left anterior superior iliac spine for introduction of the 11-mm trocar.

Third Port (5 mm, suction device)

A cutaneous incision is made 2 cm medial and superior to the right anterior superior iliac spine for introduction of the 5-mm trocar.

Fourth Port
(5 mm, monopolar round-tipped scissors)

For insertion of the 5-mm trocar, a cutaneous incision is made at a point situated at the junction of the lateral 2/3 and medial 1/3 distance between the right anterior superior iliac spine trocar and the umbilicus trocar.

> **TIP**
>
> *Pay attention to the epigastric vessels, which can be visualized by pressing the right lateral part of the abdomen.*

The operating table is moved down and backward, and the patient is placed in an extended Trendelenburg position. Steps are placed under the surgeon, and the bipolar and monopolar pedals are placed over the step. The surgeon, positioned higher than the assistant can then use the working instruments (bipolar grasper and monopolar scissors) without being restrained by the assistant holding the optic in the upper midline position.

Surgical Technique

The intestine is positioned above the promontory by gently pushing back the loops of the small bowel with the aid of the Trendelenburg position. If necessary, the cecum is dissected off the posterior peritoneum to increase its mobility and assist in the cranial displacement of the small bowel. To facilitate the left-side dissection, the sigmoid and its mesocolon are laterally displaced and fixed to the abdominal wall using a monofilament 2-0 straight needle suture.

> **TIP**
>
> *The suture needle is passed through the skin at a point lateral and cranial to the left port, placed through the appendices epiploicae of the sigmoid colon, and exited close to the entrance point. It is held in place by a Kocher clamp.*

The fixation has to be released for the left pelvic wall dissection.

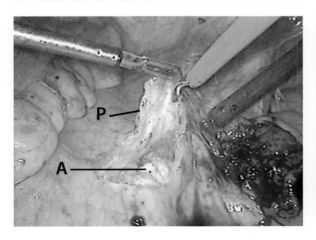

FIG. 3

Posterior peritoneal (P) incision over common iliac artery (A)

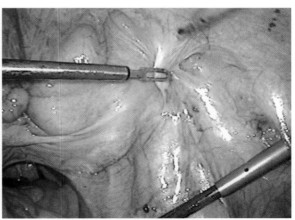

FIG. 4

Peritoneal incision extends to obliterated umbilical artery

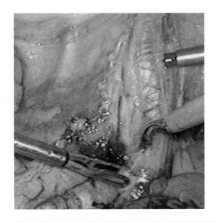

FIG. 5

Right iliac artery exposed

Transperitoneal Pelvic Lymph Node Dissection for Bladder Cancer

A standard pelvic lymphadenectomy is bilaterally performed, using a "split and roll" technique. Dissecting the lymphatic package upward, from the junction of the femoral canal up to the level of the bifurcation of the

common iliac artery, allows for an avascular plane of dissection and facilitates the laparoscopic maneuvers.

TIP

Due to technical ease, right-handed surgeons begin the dissection with the right side of the lymphadenectomy.

A posterior peritoneal incision is made over the right common iliac artery, and the medial peritoneal leaf is lifted to better expose the artery (Fig. 3).

TIP

It is important to always place traction on the peritoneum to facilitate dissection.

The incision follows the artery caudally to a point just lateral to the medial umbilical ligament (obliterated umbilical artery), at the level of the crossing of the vas deferens (round ligament in female patients) (Fig. 4); cranially, the incision extends to the common iliac artery (Fig. 5).

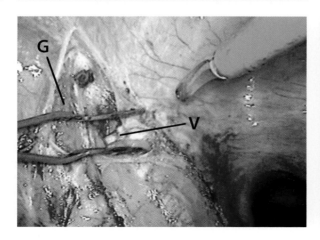

FIG. 6

Left vas (V) is coagulated and transected, and gonadal vessels (G) are laterally displaced

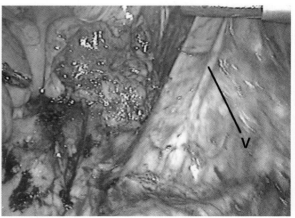

FIG. 7

"Flat" iliac vein (V)

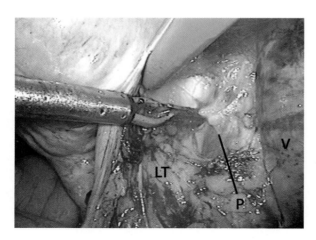

FIG. 8

Dissected tissue (LT) is swept over the psoas (P) to the obturator fossa; Iliac vein (V)

The ureters are bilaterally dissected, clipped, and displaced upward. In women, the infundibulopelvic ligament, along with the ovarian vessels, has been previously ligated and divided (see Chap. 7). The gonadal vessels are laterally displaced and preserved in the male,

and the vas deferens (round ligament) is coagulated and transected (Fig. 6).

The genitofemoral nerve, which is the lateral limit of the node dissection, should be identified and preserved as it courses over the right iliopsoas muscle. The right external iliac vessels are medially retracted, and the fascia overlying the muscle is incised medial to the nerve. The fibroareolar tissue is lifted off the surface of the muscle and is swept medially towards the iliac vessels.

The fibroareolar and lymphatic tissue anterior to the right external iliac artery is longitudinally divided using the monopolar scissors, and the tissue is dissected from the artery at its lateral and medial aspect. The same dissection is performed on the right external iliac vein.

> **TIP**
>
> *The external iliac vein appears flat at the standard pneumoperitoneum pressure (12 mmHg). To improve visualization, the pressure can be decreased to allow re-distention of the vessel (Fig.7).*

The dissection is then carried down behind the iliac vessels to free the lateral and medial component at-

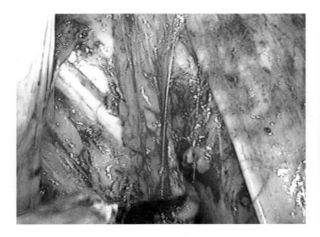

FIG. 9

Caudal limit of the dissection

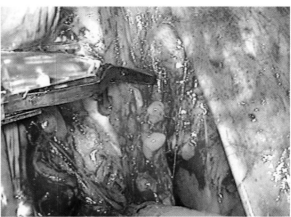

FIG. 10

Clip at nodal package

tached at their base. The vessels are carefully displaced laterally, and the lateral component of the fibroareolar and lymphatic tissue is swept under the vessels and along the psoas muscle and pelvic sidewall to the obturator fossa (Fig. 8).

At the *caudal limit* of the dissection, in the angle between Cooper's ligament and the inferior aspect of the external iliac vein (Fig. 9), the nodal package is double-clipped (Ligaclip II ML) and transected to reduce the occurrence of lymphocele (Fig. 10).

> **TIP**
>
> *The node of Cloquet, representing the distal limit of the dissection at this level, is dissected at the junction of the femoral canal (Fig. 11).*

A circumflex iliac vein usually runs to the external iliac vein at this location, and it can be ligated and divided if necessary.

The obturator nerve is visualized deep to the external iliac vein (Fig. 12), and the lymphatic package is then carefully mobilized off the obturator neurovascular bundle.

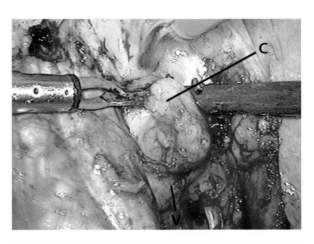

FIG. 11

Node of Cloquet (C); Accessory obturator vein (V) under the node

> **TIP**
>
> *Care must be taken not to injure the obturator nerve (Fig. 13a,b).*

The dissection at this level is bordered by the obliterated umbilical artery and lateral bladder wall, which is the *medial limit* of the dissection. Small lymphatic vessels are clipped with Ligaclip II ML.

The dissection progresses cephalad to the bifurcation of the iliac vessels, and the hypogastric artery, which is the *posterior limit* of the dissection, is visualized (Fig. 14).

The lymphatic tissue is gently stripped of the hypogastric artery (Fig. 15), and care must be taken not to injure the hypogastric vein (Fig. 16).

The dissected package is then clipped (XL Hem-o-lok clips) and transected. The specimen is removed through the left 11-mm port after being placed into a bag (Endo-Catch). The same dissection is done on the left side.

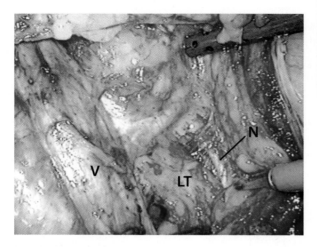

FIG. 12

Obturator nerve (N) visualized medial to the external iliac vein (V); Lymphatic tissue (LT)

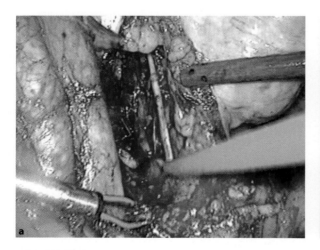

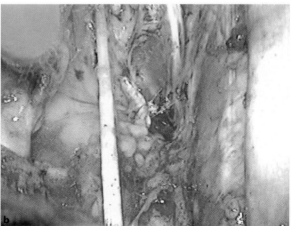

FIG. 13

a Obturator fossa. **b** Obturator artery and nerve

Transperitoneal Pelvic Lymph Node Dissection for Prostate Cancer

A standard pelvic lymphadenectomy is bilaterally performed using a "split and roll" technique. A posterior peritoneal incision is made over the right common iliac artery, and the medial peritoneal leaf is lifted to better expose the artery (Fig. 3).

> **TIP**
>
> *It is important to always place traction on the peritoneum to facilitate dissection.*

The incision follows the artery caudally to a point just medial to the medial umbilical ligament (obliterated umbilical artery), at the level of the crossing of the vas deferens (Fig. 4). Cranially, the incision extends to the bifurcation of the iliac vessels (*cephalad limit* of the dissection) (Fig. 5). The ureter is exposed at the location where it crosses the iliac artery, and it is then medially displaced together with the medial leaf of the posterior peritoneum.

The gonadal vessels are laterally displaced and preserved, and the vas deferens is coagulated and transected (Fig. 6).

The genitofemoral nerve, which is the *lateral limit* of the node dissection, should be identified and preserved as it courses over the right iliopsoas muscle. The right external iliac vessels are medially retracted, and the fas-

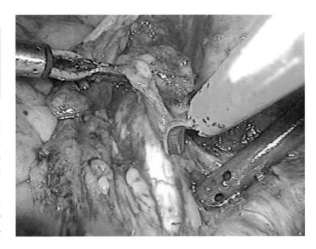

FIG. 14
Hypogastric artery

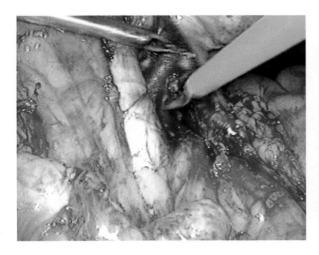

FIG. 15
Hypogastric artery dissected

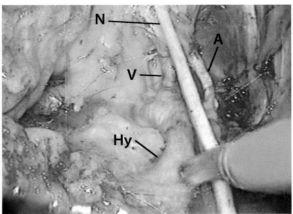

FIG. 16
Hypogastric vein (Hy); Obturator vein (V); Nerve (N); Artery (A)

cia overlying the muscle is incised medial to the nerve. The fibroareolar tissue is lifted off the surface of the muscle and is swept medially towards the iliac vessels.

The fibroareolar and lymphatic tissue anterior to the right external iliac artery is longitudinally divided using the monopolar scissors, and the tissue is dissected from the artery at its lateral and medial aspect.

The same dissection is performed on the right external iliac vein.

> **TIP**
>
> *The external iliac vein appears flat at the standard pneumoperitoneum pressure (12 mmHg). To improve visualization, the pressure can be decreased to allow re-distention of the vessel (Fig. 7).*

The dissection is then carried down behind the iliac vessels to free the lateral and medial component attached at their base. The vessels are carefully displaced laterally, and the lateral component of the fibroareolar and lymphatic tissue is swept under the vessels and along the psoas muscle and pelvic sidewall to the obturator fossa (Fig. 8).

At the *caudal limit* of the dissection, in the angle between Cooper's ligament and the inferior aspect of the external iliac vein (Fig. 9), the nodal package is double-clipped (Ligaclip II ML) and transected to reduce the occurrence of lymphocele (Fig. 10).

> **TIP**
>
> *The node of Cloquet, representing the distal limit of the dissection at this level, is dissected at the junction of the femoral canal (Fig. 11).*

A circumflex iliac vein usually runs to the external iliac vein at this location, and it can be ligated and divided if necessary.

The obturator nerve is visualized deep to the external iliac vein (Fig. 12), and the lymphatic package is then carefully mobilized off the obturator neurovascular bundle.

> **TIP**
>
> *Care must be taken not to injure the obturator nerve (Fig 13a,b).*

The dissection at this level is bordered by the obliterated umbilical artery, which is the *medial limit* of the dissection and should be preserved. Small lymphatic vessels are clipped with Ligaclip II ML.

The dissection progresses cephalad to the bifurcation of the iliac vessels, and the hypogastric artery, which is the *posterior limit* of the dissection, is visualized (Fig. 14). The lymphatic tissue is gently stripped of the hypogastric artery (Fig. 15), and care must be taken not to injure the hypogastric vein (Fig. 16).

The dissected package is then clipped (XL Hem-o-lok clips) and transected. The specimen is removed through the left 11-mm port after being placed into a bag (Endo-Catch). The same dissection is done on the left side.

Postoperative Considerations

After surgery, the patient should be treated as described in Chaps. 6 and 7.

Suggested Readings

Lymphadenectomy for Bladder Cancer

1. Haber GP, Gill IS: Laparoscopic radical cystectomy for cancer: oncological outcomes at up to 5 years. BJU Int 2007 Jul; 100(1):137–142.
2. Stein JP, Penson DF: Radical cystectomy with extended lymphadenectomy: evaluating separate package versus en bloc submission for node positive bladder cancer. J Urol 2007 Nov; 52(5):1347–55.
3. Stein JP: Lymphadenectomy in bladder cancer: how high is "high enough"? Urol Oncol 2006 Jul–Aug; 24(4):349–355.

4. Finelli A, Gill IS: Laparoscopic extended pelvic lymphadenectomy for bladder cancer: technique and initial outcomes. J Urol 2004 Nov; 172(5 Pt 1):1809–1812.

5. Stein JP, Skinner DG: The role of lymphadenectomy in high-grade invasive bladder cancer. Urol Clin North Am 2005 May; 32(2):187–197.

6. Bochner BH, Herr HW: Impact of separate versus en bloc pelvic lymph node dissection on the number of lymph nodes retrieved in cystectomy specimens. J Urol 2001 Dec; 166(6):2295–2296.

7. Vieweg J, Gschwend JE: Pelvic lymph node dissection can be curative in patients with node positive bladder cancer. J Urol 1999 Feb; 161(2):449–454.

Lymphadenectomy for Prostate Cancer

1. Heidenreich A, Ohlmann CH: Anatomical extent of pelvic lymphadenectomy in patients undergoing radical prostatectomy. Eur Urol 2007 Jul; 52(1):29–37.

2. Lattouf JB, Beri A: Laparoscopic extended pelvic lymph node dissection for prostate cancer: description of the surgical technique and initial results. Eur Urol 2007 Nov; 52(5):1347–55.

3. Touijer K, Rabbani F: Standard vs limited pelvic lymph node dissection for prostate cancer in patients with a predicted probability of nodal metastasis greater than 1%. J Urol 2007 July; 178(1):120–124.

4. Wyler SF, Sulser T: Laparoscopic extended pelvic lymph node dissection for high-risk prostate cancer. Urology 2006 Oct; 68(4):883–887.

5. Häcker A, Jeschke S: Detection of pelvic lymph node metastases in patients with clinically localized prostate cancer: comparison of [18F] fluorocholine positron emission tomography-computerized tomography and laparoscopic radioisotope guided sentinel lymph node dissection. J Urol 2006 Nov; 176(5):2014–8; discussion 2018–2019.

6. Stone NN, Stock RG: Laparoscopic pelvic lymph node dissection for prostate cancer: comparison of the extended and modified techniques. J Urol 1997 Nov; 158(5):1891–1894.

Section III

Laparoscopic Surgery for Benign Urological Disorders

Chapter 9

Transperitoneal Laparoscopic Pyeloplasty

Contents

Introduction

Open pyeloplasty, once the reference standard for the correction of ureteropelvic junction (UPJ) obstruction, has fallen out of favor despite long-term success rates due to the postoperative morbidity associated with open flank surgery. Laparoscopic dismembered flap pyeloplasty is now a viable alternative for patients with UPJ obstruction, with the benefits of shorter hospital stays, reduced postoperative pain, and faster convalescence. The laparoscopic approach is capable of addressing various clinical situations of UPJ obstruction, and depending on expertise level, has proved to be equally efficacious in treating scarred, obstructed UPJ that had failed open surgery.

Preoperative Preparation

Before a patient consents to a laparoscopic pyeloplasty, it is important to discuss the specific risks of the surgery, including the potential need to convert to the traditional open operation if difficulties arise.

The patient is admitted to the hospital the day before the surgery for bowel preparation, which includes 2 L of Colopeg® (1 envelope/L) p.o. and a Fleet® enema. Fasting starts at midnight before surgery. Patients also receive antibiotic prophylaxis with a single preoperative dose of intravenous second-generation cephalosporin, unless they are allergic to penicillin. Blood type and crossmatch are determined.

Patient Positioning and Initial Preparation

The patient is initially positioned supine for intravenous access, the induction of general anesthesia, and endotracheal intubation. An orogastric tube is placed and the stomach decompressed to avoid puncture during trocar placement and to allow additional space during abdominal insufflation. An 18Fr Foley catheter with 10 mL in the balloon is introduced for decompression of the bladder. During skin preparation, the entire flank and abdomen are included in case conversion to an open procedure is required. The umbilicus is placed over the break in the operating table, and the patient is positioned in a modified lateral decubitus position.

> **TIP**
>
> *For left-side pyeloplasty, the patient is placed in a strict lateral decubitus position.*

The table can be flexed as needed or an inflatable balloon is positioned under the patient at the level of the umbilicus. Padding is used to support the buttocks and torso, and all potential pressure points are cushioned.

An axillary roll is placed to prevent brachial plexus injury, and the arms are positioned as far away from the trunk as possible so as not to disturb the movement of the operative team. The patient is held in position with strips of cloth tape (Fig. 1a,b).

The surgeon operates from the abdominal side of the patient, and the first assistant is placed caudally to the surgeon. The laparoscopic cart is positioned at the back of the patient's chest, with the operative team facing the video monitor. The instruments table is positioned behind the operative team, and the assistant is positioned higher than the surgeon to prevent instruments from conflicting (Fig. 2a–c).

Trocars and Laparoscopic Instruments

Right-side pyeloplasty:
- 2 × 11 mm (optic 0° and bipolar grasper)
- 3 × 5 mm (monopolar scissors, suction device, and liver retractor grasper)

Left-side pyeloplasty:
- 2 × 11 mm (optic 0° and bipolar grasper)
- 2 × 5 mm (monopolar scissors and suction device)

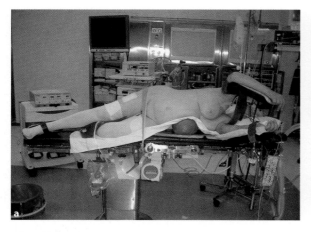
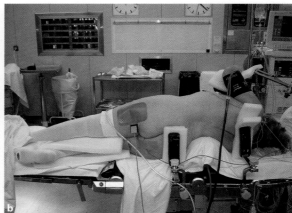

FIG. 1

a Patient position. **b** Padding

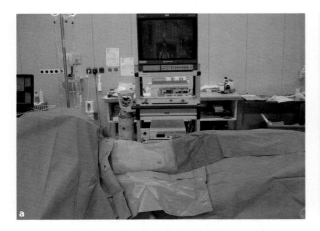

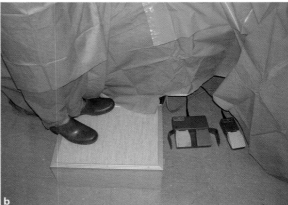

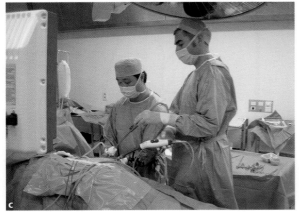

FIG. 2

a Patient and laparoscopic cart. **b** Steps below assistant.
c Instruments table behind operative team

- Monopolar round-tipped scissors, bipolar grasper, liver retractor grasper, 5-mm suction device, needle drivers (2), and 10-mm laparoscopic optic 0°

Access and Port Placement

Four ports are generally enough to perform the procedure, although a fifth port may be used for liver retraction in those cases of secondary reconstruction with long length of proximal ureteral stenosis, where the right kidney must be fully mobilized (Fig. 3). Before the introduction of the trocars, the abdomen is insufflated using a Veress needle.

TIP

In case of previous surgery, the Veress needle is not inserted, and an open access procedure is done for the placement of the first trocar.

Veress Needle

A cutaneous incision is made two fingerbreadths below the costal margin arch in the midaxillary line, lateral to the ipsilateral rectus muscle (see Chap. 1, Veress Needle

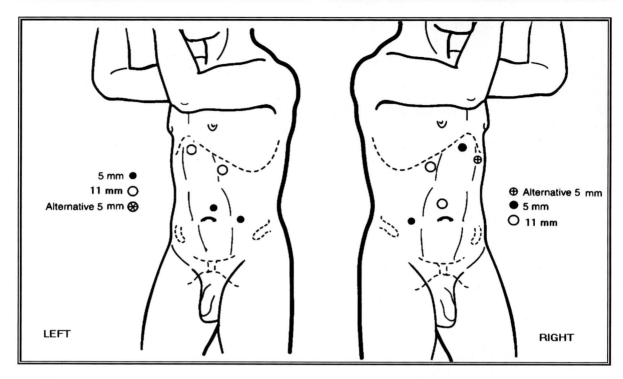

FIG. 3

Access and port placement (This figure was published in Wein: Campbell-Walsh Urology, 9th ed., Copyright Elsevier)

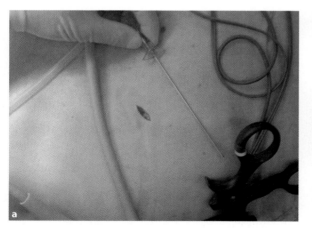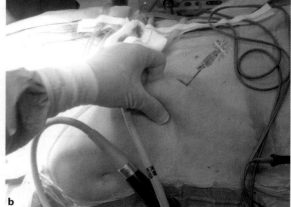

FIG. 4

a Veress needle at the costal margin arch. **b** Veress needle inserted

Introduction). The needle is introduced through the incision (Fig. 4a,b).

TIP

The skin incision should be 50% larger than the diameter of the 11-mm trocar.

First Port (11 mm, optic 0°)

Once pneumoperitoneum is established, the Veress needle is removed, and the 11-mm trocar is introduced through the same incision, perpendicularly to the abdominal wall (Fig. 5).

TIP

Pneumoperitoneum is established with an intra-abdominal pressure higher than 10 mmHg.

The optic is introduced through the device, and the abdomen is then inspected for any injury due to insertion of the Veress needle or the trocar, and to identify adhesions in areas where the secondary ports will be placed. The insufflator line is then connected to the trocar.

Second Port (5 mm, monopolar round-tipped scissors)

The triangulation rule must be followed for the placement of the trocars as the body habitus is different for each patient. Four fingerbreadths should be between the optic trocar and the working trocars (Fig. 6), and five fingerbreadths should be between the working trocars (Fig. 7a,b).

TIP

The 5-mm port is usually reserved for the most skilled hand, as the movements of the working instruments inside the smaller ports must be precise.

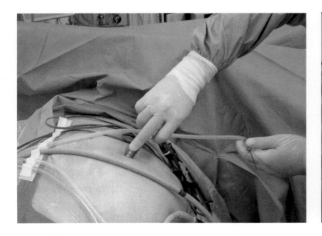

FIG. 5
Perpendicular introduction of the trocar

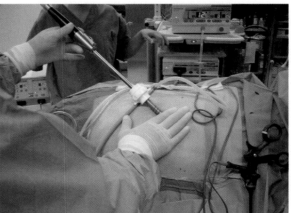

FIG. 6
Triangulation rule, four fingers

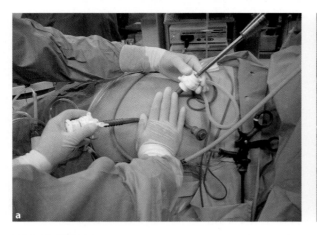

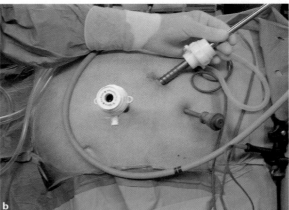

FIG. 7

a Triangulation rule, five fingers. b Ports in place

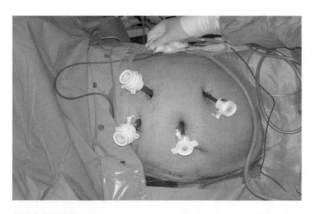

FIG. 8

Left-side ports in position

Third Port (11 mm, bipolar grasper)

The triangulation rule must be followed as above (Fig. 7a,b).

Fourth Port (5 mm, suction device)

A cutaneous incision is made approximately midline between the umbilicus trocar and the anterior superior iliac spine on the side of the procedure for the introduction of the 5-mm trocar.

Final Position of the Ports

The ports are tied to the skin with Vicryl 2-0 to prevent accidental removal.

Surgical Technique

Colon Mobilization

A traditional Anderson-Hynes dismembered pyeloplasty is the usual preferred technique for patients who have a large renal pelvis, a high ureteral insertion, or a posterior crossing vessel at the ureteropelvic junction. For a left pyeloplasty, the plane between the descending colon and the underlying Gerota's fascia is developed to allow the colon to fall medially (Fig. 9a,b). On the right, the ascending colon is mobilized and dissected from the underlying Gerota's fascia.

TIP

The lateral attachments of the kidney to the abdominal wall should not be freed at this time to avoid the kidney falling medially into the operating field.

TIP

In thin patients, a transmesocolic approach can be used, and the colon is not mobilized.

Colon mobilization continues caudally to the common iliac vessels.

Identification of the Ureter and Ureteropelvic Junction (UPJ)

Gerota's fascia is carefully incised at the level of the lower pole of the kidney for the dissection of the ureteropelvic junction and potential associated crossing vessels. Otherwise, the ureter can be searched inferior to the lower pole of the kidney and followed to the ureteropelvic junction. The Gerota's fatty tissue at the level of the lower pole is incised and lifted to locate the psoas muscle.

TIP

The correct maneuver to expose the psoas muscle is the continuous upper movement of the laparoscopic instruments to lift the fatty tissue.

The psoas is followed to expose the gonadal vessels and the ureter just lateral and deep to these vessels.

TIP

In case of previous surgery or difficulty in finding the ureter, it should be dissected in a lower location.

The ureter is carefully dissected from the gonadal vessels, and attachments between these structures are released with the aid of monopolar scissors.

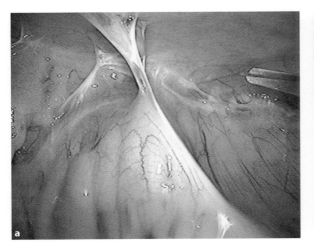 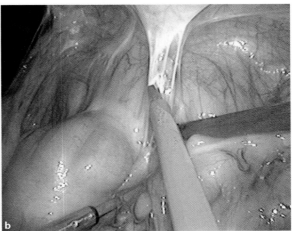

FIG. 9

a Colon adhesions to peritoneum. **b** Plane between colon and Gerota's fascia

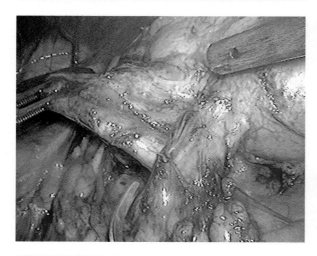

FIG. 10
Pelvic junction and crossing vessel

> **TIP**
>
> *Care must be taken not to excise too much renal pelvis, especially when resecting along its lateral aspect to avoid anastomosis tension.*

The ureter wall is opened longitudinally and spatulated for about 1.5 to 2.0 cm along its *lateral* margin (Fig. 12).

> **TIP**
>
> *If no urine exits from the proximal end of the transected ureter, an intrinsically related problem is the most likely cause of the UPJ stenosis.*

> **TIP**
>
> *The ureteral blood supply is usually anteromedially located in the proximal third, medially located in the middle third, and laterally located in the distal third.*

The ureter is then lifted and, along with the visualization of the psoas muscle, followed cranially to the lower pole and to the ureteropelvic junction.

Ureteral Transection/Renal Pelvis Excision

Following identification of the ureteropelvic pathology, the pelvic junction and the renal pelvis are carefully dissected to allow mobilization of these structures (Fig. 10).

After determining that there is adequate ureteral length for the anastomosis, the ureter is transected close to the UPJ. The ureteropelvic junction is incised, and the redundant renal pelvis is *diagonally* excised from its *lateral* side (Fig. 11a–c).

Anastomosis

After proper alignment of the ureter and renal pelvis, the first Vicryl 4-0 suture is placed through the apex of the "V" in the spatulated ureter and through the tip of the inferior renal pelvic flap (Fig. 13a,b).

> **TIP**
>
> *The suture is placed from the outside of the lumen of the ureter to the inside of the lumen of the renal pelvis.*

Tying of the first suture advances and reduces the tension on the anastomosis.

> **TIP**
>
> *In case of anastomosis tension, the ureter can be further freed distally to allow for cranial mobilization.*

The needle is then passed under the ureter to perform the *posterior* side of the anastomosis.

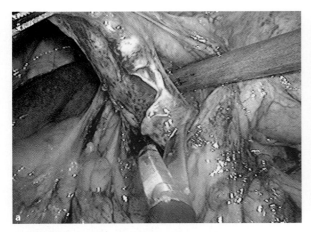

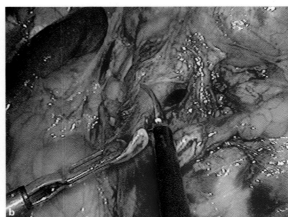

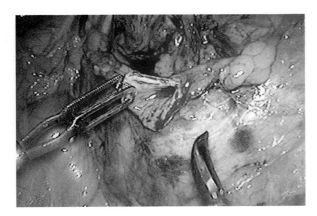

FIG. 11

a Ureteropelvic junction incision. b Redundant pelvis diagonally incised. c Redundant pelvis excised

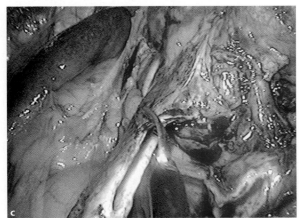

FIG. 12

Ureteral spatulation along lateral margin

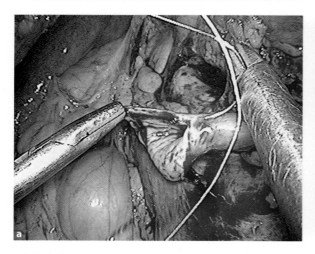

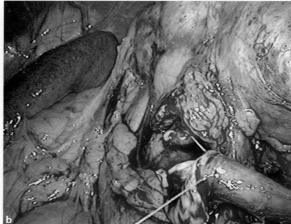

FIG. 13

a Suture placed at ureter. **b** Initial ureteropelvic suture

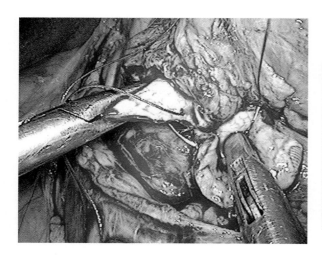

A watertight running suture is done following a cephalad course.

> **TIP**
>
> *The initial suture at the renal pelvis is placed from the outside to the inside of the lumen; the suture is then introduced from the inside of the lumen of the ureter and again to the outside of the lumen of the renal pelvis (Fig. 14). To avoid the crossing of the suture during this stage, the standing part of the thread is positioned in the center of the anastomosis facing the renal pelvis.*

FIG. 14

Posterior side of the anastomosis

After completing the posterior anastomosis (Fig. 15), the knot is tied, and a double J stent is introduced.

Stenting

> **TIP**
>
> *The backside of the needle is passed first when moving the needle under the ureter to perform the posterior side of the anastomosis.*

A straight tip guide wire introduced through the working 11-mm port is inserted into the ureter and down to the bladder (Fig. 16). A 7Fr double-pigtail stent (26–30 cm long) is placed in an antegrade fashion over the

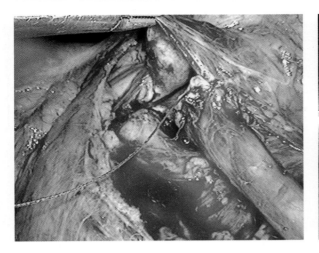

FIG. 15
Posterior anastomosis completed

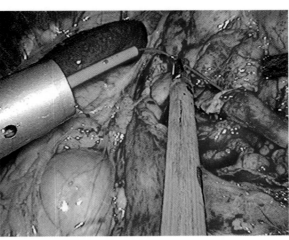

FIG. 16
Guide wire inserted

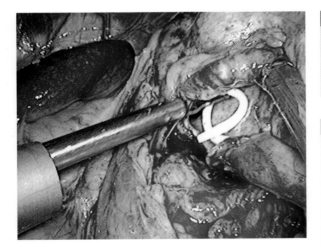

FIG. 17
Proximal part of stent placed into the renal pelvis

> **TIP**
>
> *The guide wire and the proximal ureter should be aligned along the same axis to facilitate wire introduction.*

> **TIP**
>
> *Approximation of the 11-mm port close to the lumen of the ureter facilitates stent introduction. The visualization of a reflux of methylene blue instilled into the bladder at the ureterotomy site can be used to verify the correct placement of the stent in the bladder.*

Alternatively, a nephroureteral catheter is inserted retrogradely through a thin renal parenchyma overlying a calyx and is exteriorized while the distal part is inserted into the ureter.

The *anterior anastomosis* is then performed (Fig. 18). A watertight cranially oriented running suture is placed from the outside of the lumen of the renal pelvis to the

guide wire into the bladder, and following removal of the guide wire, the proximal part of the stent is placed into the renal pelvis (Fig. 17).

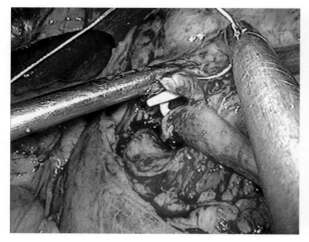

FIG. 18

Anterior anastomosis

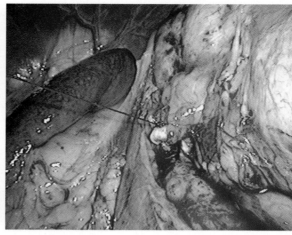

FIG. 19

Final result

inside of the lumen of the ureter, and the knot is tied (Fig. 19).

A Penrose drain is introduced through the 11-mm port, positioned adjacent to the repair, and exited through the most caudal port. The aponeurosis of the 11-mm port is closed with a Dexon II HGU-46 suture, and the skin is closed with running intradermic Monocryl 3-0. The drain is fixed to the skin with Flexidene 2-0, and the skin incisions are closed with Opsite® dressing.

Postoperative Considerations

A short hospitalization is associated with laparoscopic pyeloplasty. The Foley catheter is removed on the second postoperative day, and the Penrose drain is usually removed before discharge. The double-J stent is left indwelling for six weeks, and objective assessment of the repair is done with diuretic nuclear renography after a three months' follow-up.

Suggested Readings

1. Williams B, Tareen B: Pathophysiology and treatment of ureteropelvic junction obstruction. Curr Urol Rep 2007 Mar; 8(2):111–117.

2. Stein RJ, Gill IS: Comparison of surgical approaches to ureteropelvic junction obstruction: endopyeloplasty versus endopyelotomy versus laparoscopic pyeloplasty. Curr Urol Rep 2007 Mar; 8(2):140–149.

3. Castillo OA, Vitagliano G: Transmesocolic pyeloplasty: experience of a single center. J Endourol 2007 Apr; 21(4):415–418.

4. Simforoosh N: Laparoscopic management of ureteropelvic junction obstruction by division of anterior crossing vein and cephalad relocation of anterior crossing artery. J Endourol 2005 Sep; 19(7):827–830.

Chapter 10

Transperitoneal Laparoscopic Donor Nephrectomy

Contents

Introduction

Laparoscopic living donor nephrectomy has become the standard procedure for renal transplantation. The laparoscopic technique is less invasive for the donor, allowing lower postoperative analgesic requirements and a faster return to daily activities. Concerns about adequate length of the right renal vein have resulted in more laparoscopic donor nephrectomies being performed on the left side, conflicting with the principle of leaving the donor with the best kidney. Although right nephrectomies are not more technically challenging than left nephrectomies, the short length of the right renal vein restrains the routine use of the right kidney for transplantation purposes. Preservation of the maximum length of the right renal vein continues to be a challenge for the surgeon, and the technique described utilizes a modified Endo GIA™ 30 Universal stapler for this purpose.

Preoperative Preparation

Before a patient consents to a laparoscopic nephrectomy, it is important to discuss the specific risks of the surgery, including the potential need to convert to the traditional open operation if difficulties arise.

The patient is admitted to the hospital the day before the surgery for bowel preparation, which includes 2 L of Colopeg® (1 envelope/L) p.o. and a Fleet® enema. Fasting starts at midnight before surgery. Thromboprophylaxis is implemented with good hydration, placement of compressive elastic stockings on the lower extremities, and low-molecular-weight heparin. Enoxaparin (Clexane®, Lovenox®) 40 mg sc 1 × day or nadroparin (Flaxiparine®, Fraxiparin®) 0.6 mL sc 1 × day is initiated on day 1 after the surgery and continued daily until the patient is discharged from the hospital. In selected cases, the treatment is continued for 30 days after the procedure. Patients also receive antibiotic prophylaxis with a single preoperative dose of intravenous second-generation cephalosporin, unless they are allergic to penicillin. Blood type and crossmatch are determined.

Patient Positioning and Initial Preparation

The patient is initially positioned supine for intravenous access, the induction of general anesthesia, and endotracheal intubation. An orogastric tube is placed and the stomach decompressed to avoid puncture during trocar placement and to allow additional space during abdominal insufflation. An 18Fr Foley catheter with 10 mL in the balloon is introduced for decompression of the bladder. During skin preparation, the entire flank and abdomen are included in case conversion to an open procedure is required. The umbilicus is placed over the break in the operating table, and the patient is positioned in a modified lateral decubitus position.

TIP

For left-side nephrectomy, the patient is placed in a strict lateral decubitus position.

The table can be flexed as needed or an inflatable balloon is positioned under the patient at the level of the umbilicus. Padding is used to support the buttocks and torso, and all potential pressure points are cushioned. An axillary roll is placed to prevent brachial plexus injury, and the arms should be positioned as far away from the trunk as possible so as not to disturb the movement of the operative team. The patient is held in position with strips of cloth tape (Fig. 1a,b).

The surgeon operates from the abdominal side of the patient, and the first assistant is placed caudally to the surgeon. The laparoscopic cart is positioned at the back of the patient's chest, with the operative team facing the video monitor. The instruments table is positioned behind the operative team, and the assistant is positioned on steps to prevent instruments from conflicting (Fig. 2a–c).

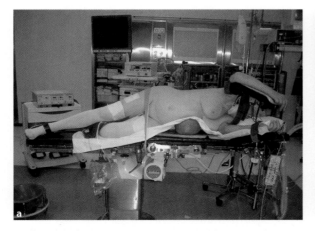
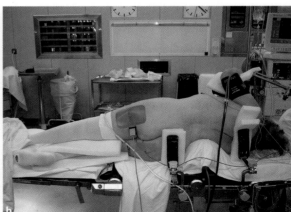

FIG. 1
a Patient position. **b** Padding

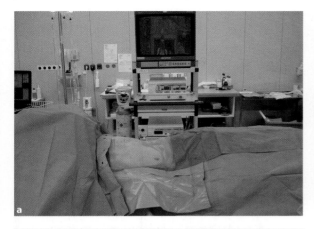

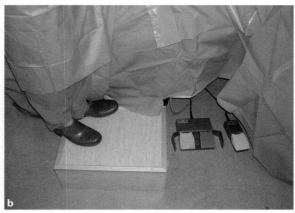

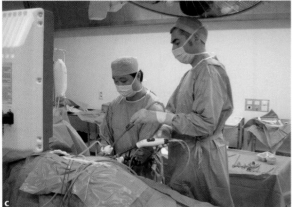

FIG. 2

a Patient and laparoscopic cart. **b** Steps below assistant.
c Instruments table behind operative team

Trocars and Laparoscopic Instruments

Right-side nephrectomy:
- 1 × 11 mm (optic 0°)
- 1 × 12 mm (Endo GIA and bipolar grasper)
- 3 × 5 mm (monopolar scissors, suction device, and liver retractor grasper)

Left-side nephrectomy:
- 2 × 11 mm (optic 0°, bipolar grasper, and 10-mm clip applier)
- 2 × 5 mm (monopolar scissors and suction device)

- Monopolar round-tipped scissors, bipolar grasper, liver retractor grasper, 5-mm suction device, needle drivers (2), 10-mm laparoscopic optic 0°, 10-mm clip applier (non-disposable), and Multifire Endo GIA™ 30 stapler

Access and Port Placement

Four ports are generally enough to perform the procedure, although a fifth trocar may be necessary for liver retraction during right-side nephrectomy (Fig. 3). Be-

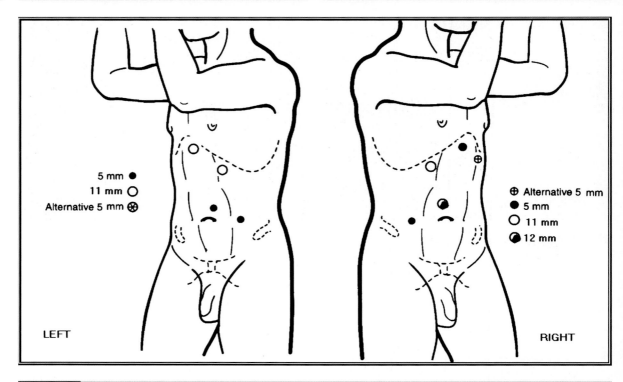

FIG. 3

Access and port placement (This figure was published in Wein: Campbell-Walsh Urology, 9th ed., Copyright Elsevier)

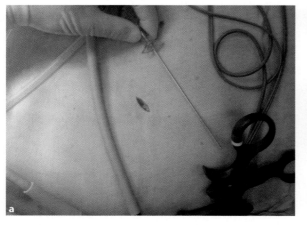

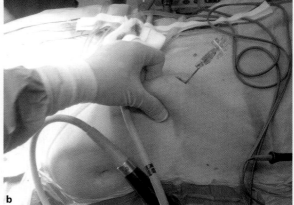

FIG. 4

a Cutaneous incision below costal margin. b Insertion of Veress needle

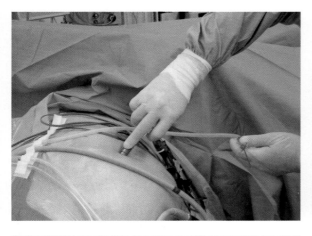

FIG. 5

Perpendicular introduction of the trocar

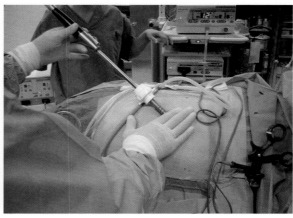

FIG. 6

Triangulation rule, four fingers

fore trocars are placed, the abdomen is insufflated using a Veress needle.

> **TIP**
>
> *In case of previous surgery, the Veress needle is not inserted, and an open access procedure is done for the placement of the first trocar.*

Veress Needle

A cutaneous incision is made two fingerbreadths below the costal margin arch, at the level of the lateral border of the rectus muscle (Fig. 4a,b).

> **TIP**
>
> *The skin incision should be 50% larger than the diameter of the 11 mm trocar.*

The Veress needle is introduced through the incision (see Chap. 1, Veress Needle Introduction).

First Port (11 mm, optic 0°)

Once pneumoperitoneum is established, the Veress needle is removed, and the 11-mm trocar is introduced through the same incision, perpendicularly to the abdominal wall (Fig. 5).

> **TIP**
>
> *Pneumoperitoneum is established with an intra-abdominal pressure higher than 10 mmHg.*

The optic is introduced through the device, and the abdomen is then inspected for any injury due to insertion of the Veress needle or the trocar, and to identify adhesions in areas where the secondary ports will be placed. The insufflator line is then connected to the port.

Second Port

- For a left-side nephrectomy: 11 mm (10-mm clip applier and bipolar grasper)
- For a right-side nephrectomy: 5 mm (monopolar round-tipped scissors)

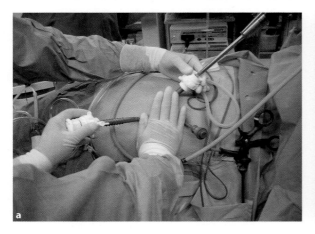

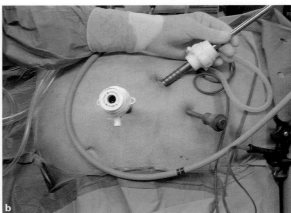

FIG. 7
a Triangulation rule, five fingers. b Ports in place

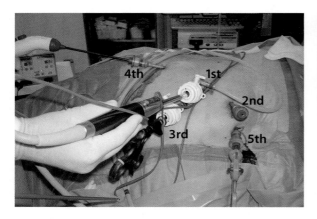

FIG. 8
Right-side ports

> **TIP**
>
> *The 5-mm port is usually reserved for the most skilled hand, because the movements of the working instruments inside the smaller ports must be precise.*

Third Port

- For a left-side nephrectomy: 5 mm (monopolar round-tipped scissors)
- For a right-side nephrectomy: 12 mm (Multifire Endo GIA 30 stapler and bipolar grasper)

The triangulation rule must be followed as above.

Fourth Port (5 mm, suction device)

A cutaneous incision is made approximately midline between the umbilicus trocar and the anterior superior iliac spine on the side of the procedure for the introduction of the 5-mm trocar.

The triangulation rule must be followed for the placement of the trocars as the body habitus is different for each patient. Four fingerbreadths should be between the optic trocar and the working trocars (Fig. 6), and five fingerbreadths should be between the working trocars (Fig. 7a,b).

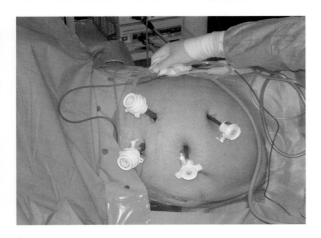

FIG. 9
Left-side ports

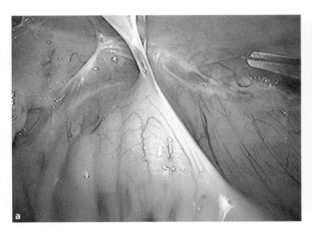

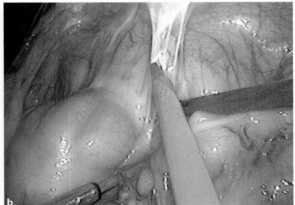

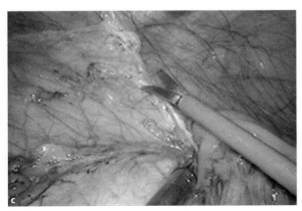

FIG. 10
a Colon attachments to abdominal wall. b Release of the colon attachments to abdominal wall. c Colon is dissected from Gerota's fascia (Gerota is not freed from abdominal wall)

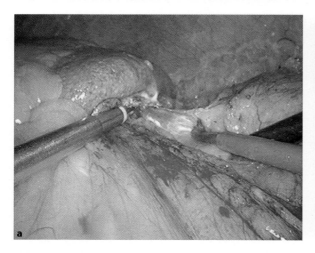 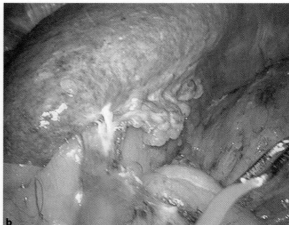

FIG. 11

a Spleen is released from kidney. **b** En bloc spleen dissection

Fifth Port (5 mm, liver retractor grasper)

A cutaneous incision is made approximately two fingerbreadths below the level of the second port for introduction of a 5-mm port in case a liver retraction is performed during a right-side nephrectomy (Fig. 8).

Final Position of the Ports

See Figures 8 and 9.

The ports are finally tied to the skin with Vicryl 2-0 to prevent accidental removal.

Surgical Technique

Colon Mobilization

For a *left-side nephrectomy*, the plane between the descending colon and the underlying Gerota's fas-

cia is developed to allow the colon to fall medially (Fig. 10a–c).

> **TIP**
>
> *The lateral attachments of Gerota's fascia to the abdominal wall should not be freed at this time to avoid the kidney falling medially into the operating field.*

This plane of dissection is carried out cranially. The splenorenal and lienocolic ligaments are incised, allowing the spleen and the tail of the pancreas to be separated from the upper pole of the kidney. The en bloc dissection of the colon, spleen, and pancreas must be completed for adequate exposure of the renal hilum (Fig. 11a,b).

For a *right-side nephrectomy*, the liver is cranially retracted using a grasper that is fixed to the abdominal wall (Fig. 12). The ascending colon is mobilized and dissected from the underlying Gerota's fascia. Colon mobilization continues caudally to the common iliac vessels.

Ureter and Gonadal Vessels Identification

Following the medial mobilization of the colon and mesocolon, the gonadal vessels are visualized underneath Gerota's fascia. The Gerota's fatty tissue at the level of the lower pole of the kidney is incised and lifted to locate the psoas muscle (Fig. 13).

TIP

The correct maneuver to expose the psoas muscle is the continuous upper movement of the laparoscopic instruments to lift the fatty tissue.

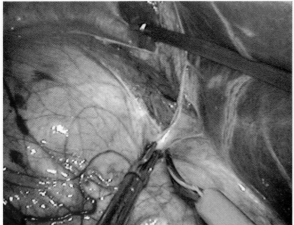

FIG. 12
Grasper retracting liver

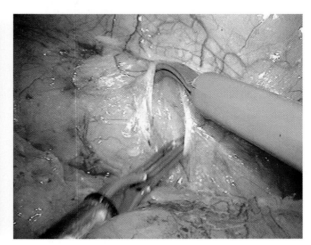

FIG. 13
Lifting of fatty tissue to expose psoas muscle

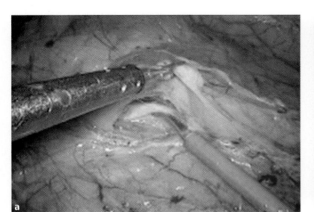

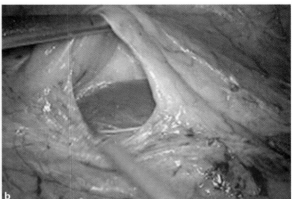

FIG. 14
a Dissection of ureter and gonadal vessels. **b** Psoas muscle

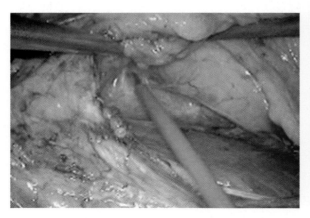

FIG. 15
Renal hilum

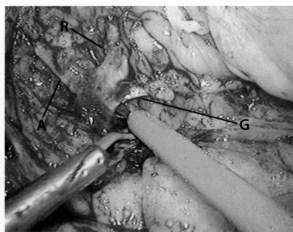

FIG. 16
Left gonadal (G), adrenal (A), and renal (R) veins

The psoas is followed to expose the ureter just lateral and deep to the gonadal vessels (Fig. 14a,b).

By tracking the cephalad course of the ureter, together with the gonadal vessels on the left side, the plane is followed up to the renal hilum (Fig. 15).

Caudally, the ureter is dissected and freed until the crossing of the iliac vessels. The ureter and gonadal vessels are not divided at this time.

Exposure and Dissection of the Renal Hilum

For a *left-side nephrectomy,* the renal vein is dissected along with the lumbar, gonadal, and adrenal veins (Fig. 16).

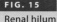
TIP

Care must be taken with: (1) the lumbar vessels that are usually located posterior and inferior to the renal vein and that cross over the renal artery and (2) the adrenal vein that usually drains at the superior margin of the renal vessel. These vessels are cut to increase the length of the renal vein.

The left renal artery is dissected and exposed posterior to the veins (Fig. 17a,b).

For a *right-side nephrectomy,* the duodenum is medially mobilized by performing a Kocher maneuver until the vena cava is clearly visualized.

TIP

For a right-side nephrectomy, the vena cava is mobilized laterally, and the left renal vein is dissected and gently displaced to expose the plane between the aorta and the inferior vena cava. The right renal artery is dissected and exposed at its origin. The aim is to attain maximal length of the donor vessel (Fig. 18).

The right renal vein is dissected at the lateral border of the vena cava.

Mobilization of the Kidney and Ureter Transection

The dissection continues cranially to the upper pole of the kidney, and the adrenal gland is separated from it.

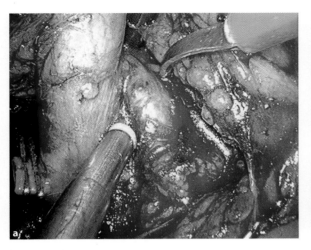

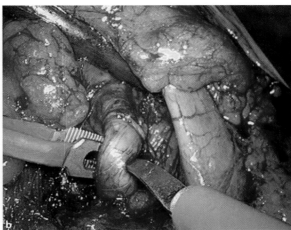

FIG. 17

a Renal artery exposed. b Renal artery dissected

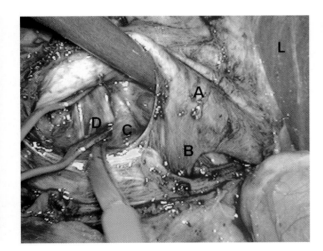

FIG. 18

Vena cava (A); Left renal vein (B); Right renal artery (C); Intercavoaortic Space (D); Liver (L)

This is accomplished by incising Gerota's fascia anteriorly just above the hilum and then carefully peeling off the Gerota's fat circumferentially above the upper pole of the kidney.

> **TIP**
>
> *At this point during the dissection, care must be taken with the short adrenal vein on the right side that drains into the inferior vena cava at its posterolateral side.*

For a *right-side nephrectomy*, superior retraction of the liver facilitates the dissection of the plane between the liver and the upper pole of the kidney (Fig. 19).

The attachments of the kidney to the posterior and lateral abdominal wall are released by blunt and sharp dissection, taking care to coagulate the bleeding vessels. Inferiorly, the ureter is ligated with one large (L) Hem-o-lok® clip applied to its most distal portion, and it is then transected to allow the kidney to be fully mobilized.

Renal Hilum Ligature

A 6–8 cm lower ilioinguinal incision is made, but the muscle attached to the peritoneum is not incised to preserve the pneumoperitoneum. A large laparoscopic bag (EndoCatch® II 15 mm, Tyco Autosuture) is introduced through the small opening of the peritoneum at the il-

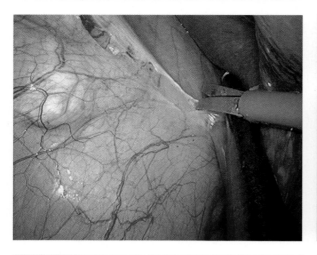

FIG. 19

Dissection plane between liver and kidney upper pole

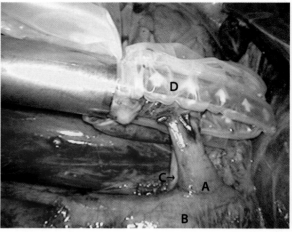

FIG. 20

Right renal vein (A); Vena cava (B); Right renal artery (C); EndoCatch metal ring (D)

ioinguinal incision. The kidney, attached only to the hilum, is placed into the bag, and the EndoCatch arm is pulled out to partially close the metal ring around the hilum (Fig. 20).

> **TIP**
>
> *A Kocher clamp is placed at the EndoCatch arm to hold the metal ring in place to prevent its opening.*

> **TIP**
>
> *The string of the EndoCatch must not be touched to avoid detachment of the bag.*

At this time, two extra-large (XL) Hem-o-lok clips are applied to the proximal portion of the renal artery without cutting it.

> **TIP**
>
> *As soon as the clip is applied to the artery, the warm ischemia begins.*

The right renal vein is gently stretched. The vein is then stapled and divided using the Multifire Endo GIA™ 30 12-mm stapler (Autosuture) introduced through the third port (12 mm). The tension on the renal vein places the row of staples on the lateral part of the vena cava, increasing the donor vein length (Fig. 21). The left renal vein is proximally clipped with two extra-large (XL) Hem-o-lok clips and then transected, leaving a 2-mm vein margin to prevent the slipping of the clips.

> **TIP**
>
> *No clips are placed at the kidney side of the renal artery and vein.*

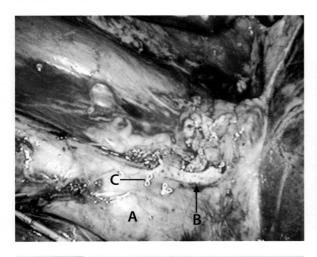

FIG. 21

Vena cava (A); Stapled cuff of vena cava (B); Loose staples (C)

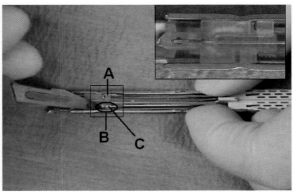

FIG. 22

Superior fixation of the pusher intact (A); Inferior fixation of the pusher sectioned (B); Clip pusher (C)

Following transection of the renal vein, the renal artery is then cut.

> **TIP**
>
> *The Multifire Endo GIA 30 stapler is used for securing and transecting the main right renal vein, but the triple staggered rows of staples of the kidney side are removed to allow for a longer donor vein (Fig. 22). The rows of staples can be individually removed using a thin needle or by cutting the fixation of the pusher at its base with a scalpel and then firing it to release the staples. The empty rows are yellow colored, facilitating the visualization of the correct side of the Endo GIA that will be applied to the renal vein (Fig. 23).*

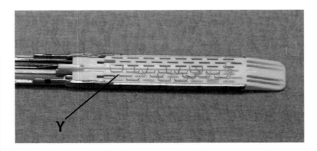

FIG. 23

Yellow colored empty rows (Y)

Kidney Extraction

Once all of the hilar vessels have been divided, a simple digital avulsion of the muscle and peritoneum around the arm of the EndoCatch opens completely the ilioinguinal incision, allowing the EndoCatch with the specimen inside to be easily removed. The kidney is then taken to the bench, where it is flushed with a preservation solution (Custodiol HTK, Tramedico).

Abdominal Closure

The abdominal wall is closed using running Vicryl 2-0 SH 1 Plus (needle ½ 21.8 mm) for the peritoneum, Vicryl 0 suture in "X" for the muscle, and a running Vicryl 1 CT Plus (needle ½ 39.9 mm) for the aponeurosis. Once the abdominal wall is closed, pneumoperitoneum is re-established, and the optic is introduced for revision of the hemostasis. A silicone Penrose drain is inserted. After evacuation of the pneumoperitoneum and removal of the trocars, the aponeurosis of the 11-mm and 12-mm ports are closed with a Dexon II HGU-46 suture. The skin incisions are closed with subcuticular Monocryl 3-0 C 423 and routinely infiltrated with 0.25% bupivacaine.

Postoperative Considerations

The nasogastric tube is removed at the end of the procedure, and the intravenous perfusion is stopped on day 1. Pain is controlled with scheduled intramuscular nonsteroidal anti-inflammatory drugs (NSAIDs) and oral analgesics. Intramuscular NSAIDs are often discontinued after 24 h. A light diet can generally be resumed on day 1 after surgery. The Foley catheter is removed on day 1 after surgery and the Penrose drain on the second postoperative day. Patients leave the hospital on the third or fourth postoperative day. Normal light activities are resumed after hospital discharge, but vigorous activities and heavy lifting are limited for at least one month after surgery.

Suggested Readings

1. Bollens R, Mikhaski D: Laparoscopic live donor right nephrectomy: a new technique to maximize the length of the renal vein using a modified Endo GIA stapler. Eur Urol 2007 May; 51(5):1326–1331.
2. Sundaram CP, Martin GL: Complications after a 5-year experience with laparoscopic donor nephrectomy: the Indiana University experience. Surg Endosc 2007 May; 21(5):724–728.
3. Breda A, Veale J: Complications of laparoscopic living donor nephrectomy and their management: the UCLA experience. Urology 2007 Jan; 69(1):49–52.
4. Chin EH, Hazzan D: Laparoscopic donor nephrectomy: intraoperative safety, immediate morbidity, and delayed complications with 500 cases. Surg Endosc 2007 Apr; 21(4):521–526.
5. Fisher PC, Montgomery JS: 200 consecutive hand assisted laparoscopic donor nephrectomies: evolution of operative technique and outcomes. J Urol 2006 Apr; 175(4):1439–1443.

Chapter 11

Hand-Assisted Bilateral Laparoscopic Intraperitoneal Nephrectomy

Contents

Introduction

Bilateral nephrectomy is occasionally indicated in symptomatic autosomal dominant polycystic kidney disease (ADPKD) patients with end-stage renal disease. These patients are subject to hypertension, hemorrhage into the renal cysts, recurrent renal calculi formation, pain, and infection. Laparoscopic hand-assisted bilateral nephrectomy provides many advantages over staged nephrectomies, including the single administration of general anesthesia. It is a safe and reliable option with lower morbidity, reduced hospitalization, and superior cosmesis when compared with open nephrectomy. Despite the technical difficulties in removing bilateral giant kidneys in a single setting, the laparoscopic hand-assisted technique is a feasible option for providing effective relief of symptoms in ADPKD patients.

Indications

- Giant symptomatic autosomal dominant polycystic kidney disease (ADPKD)
- Acquired cystic kidney disease (ACKD) and incidental renal tumors

Preoperative Preparation

Before a patient consents to a laparoscopic hand-assisted bilateral nephrectomy, it is important to discuss the specific risks of the surgery, including the potential need to convert to the traditional open operation if difficulties arise.

The patient is admitted to the hospital the night before the surgery for bowel preparation, which includes

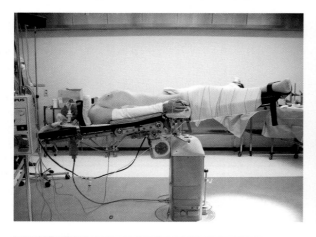

FIG. 1

Patient's position

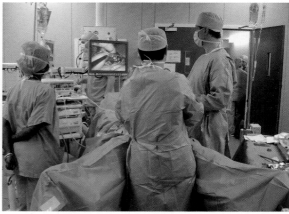

FIG. 2

Operative team's position

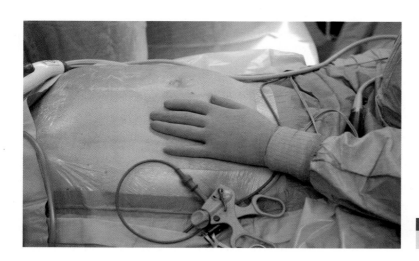

FIG. 3

Dark-colored gloves

2 L of Colopeg (1 envelope/L) p.o. and a Fleet enema. Fasting starts at midnight before surgery. Thromboprophylaxis is implemented with good hydration, placement of compressive elastic stockings on the lower extremities, and low-molecular-weight heparin. Enoxaparin (Clexane®, Lovenox®) 40 mg sc 1 × day or nadroparin (Flaxiparine®, Fraxiparin®) 0.6 mL sc 1 × day is initiated on day 1 after the surgery and continued daily until the patient is discharged from the hospital. In selected cases, the treatment is continued for 30 days after the proce-

dure. Patients also receive antibiotic prophylaxis with a single preoperative dose of intravenous second-generation cephalosporin, unless they are allergic to penicillin. Blood type and crossmatch are determined.

Patient Positioning and Initial Preparation

The surgery is performed under general anesthesia. The base of the table must be positioned below the patient's hip to avoid elevation of the abdomen while in the Trendelenburg position. The patient is placed in the supine position with the lower limbs in abduction, allowing the surgeon to be placed between the legs of the patient. The lower buttocks must be placed at the distal end of the operating table. The upper limbs are positioned alongside the body to avoid the risk of stretch injuries to the brachial plexus and to allow for free movements of the operative team (Fig. 1).

A nasogastric catheter is placed by the anesthesiologist and the stomach decompressed to avoid puncture during trocar placement and to allow additional space during extraperitoneal insufflation. The abdomen, pelvis, and genitalia are skin prepared in case conversion to an open procedure is required. An 18Fr Foley catheter with 10 mL in the balloon is introduced before the placement of the sterile drapes.

The surgeon is positioned between the patient's legs; the first assistant initially stands at the patient's left side (Fig. 2) and then moves to the right side for the left nephrectomy stage. For the right nephrectomy stage, the laparoscopic cart is placed to the right side, lateral to the patient's head, while the instruments table and the coagulation unit are positioned at the left side of the patient. For the left-side nephrectomy, the monitor is placed at the patient's left side.

Trocars and Laparoscopic Instruments

- 3×11 mm (optic 0°, scissors, suction device, and LigaSure)
- Monopolar round-tipped scissors, suction device, needle drivers (2), 10-mm laparoscopic optic 0°, LigaSure 5 mm.

> **TIP**
>
> *The surgeon uses dark-colored surgical gloves to reduce light reflection while performing the hand-assisted procedure (Fig. 3).*

Access and Port Placement

Veress Needle

A cutaneous incision is made at the level of the inferior margin of the umbilicus.

> **TIP**
>
> *The skin incision should be 50% larger than the diameter of the 11-mm trocar.*

The Veress needle is introduced through the incision (see Chap. 1, Veress Needle Introduction). The insufflation line is connected to the Veress needle, the stopcock is opened, and insufflation is initiated.

> **TIP**
>
> *It is recommended to start with low flow to avoid damage to a vital structure in case the needle is malpositioned. Switch to high flow if the pressure of insufflation is increasing at a steady and normal level and there is also a tympanic percussion of the liver area.*

First Port (11 mm, optic 0°, scissors, LigaSure)

Once pneumoperitoneum is established, the Veress needle is removed, and the 11-mm trocar is introduced through the same incision, perpendicularly to the abdominal wall.

> **TIP**
>
> *Pneumoperitoneum is established with an intra-abdominal pressure higher than 10 mmHg.*

The optic is introduced through the trocar, and the abdomen is then inspected for any injury due to insertion

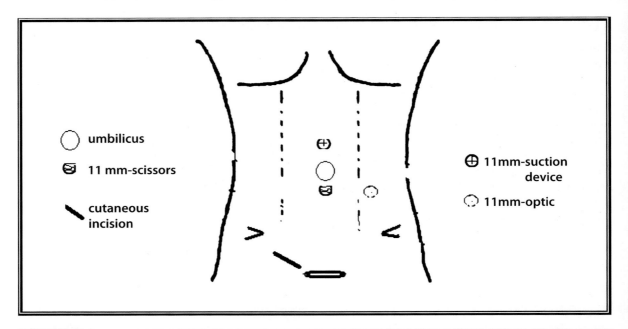

FIG. 4

Access and port placement (This figure was published in Wein: Campbell-Walsh Urology, 9th ed., Copyright Elsevier)

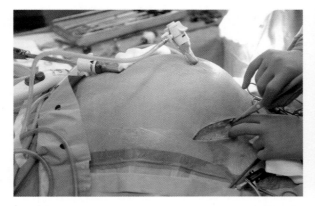

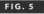

FIG. 5

Ilioinguinal cutaneous incision

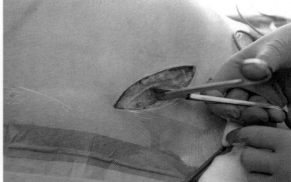

FIG. 6

Peritoneal puncture made with Mayo scissors

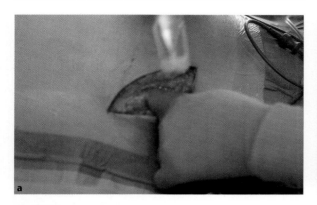 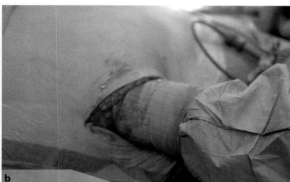

FIG. 7

a Gel applied to fingers. **b** Hand inserted

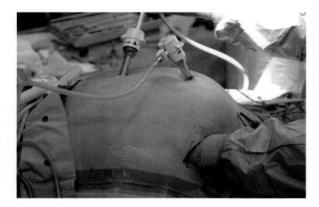

FIG. 8

Hand inside abdomen aids with trocar insertion

TIP

If a kidney graft is already in place, the hand port is medially displaced.

With the aid of Mayo scissors, a peritoneal puncture is made at the incision for the insertion of one finger (Fig. 6), and, following successive introduction of the other fingers, the full left hand is introduced (Fig. 7a, b).

TIP

Jelly is applied to the fingers to facilitate their introduction, and the hand must snugly fit into the incision to avoid air leakage.

of the Veress needle or the trocar, and to identify adhesions in areas where the secondary ports will be placed. The insufflation tubing is then connected.

Cutaneous Incision (hand introduction)

A right ilioinguinal cutaneous incision is made, and the planes are opened to expose the muscle and the peritoneum attached to it (Fig. 5).

Second Port (11 mm, optic and suction device)

A skin incision is made four fingerbreadths above the umbilicus in the midline, and an 11-mm trocar is introduced under vision and with the aid of the hand inserted into the abdominal cavity (Fig. 8).

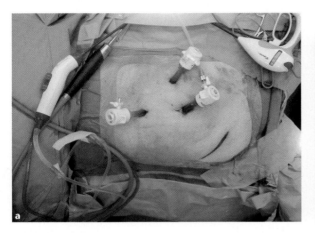
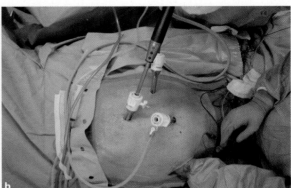

FIG. 9

a Trocars in place. **b** Trocars and hand in place

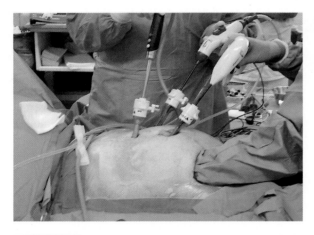

FIG. 10

Instruments in place

Third Port (11 mm, optic)

A skin incision is made four fingerbreadths to the left of the umbilicus.

> **TIP**
>
> *The incision should be 50% larger than the diameter of the 11-mm trocar.*

An 11-mm trocar is introduced under vision and with the aid of the hand inserted into the abdominal cavity (Fig. 9a,b).

Surgical Technique

Sequence of dissection:
- 1. Right kidney lower pole
- 2. Right kidney upper pole
- 3. Left kidney lower pole
- 4. Left kidney upper pole

> **TIP**
>
> *This dissection sequence will avoid excessive enlarging of the abdominal cavity incision, reducing the possibility of air leakage.*

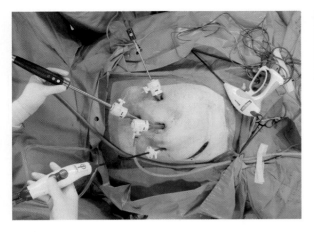

FIG. 11

Change of position of instruments for bilateral ureterectomy

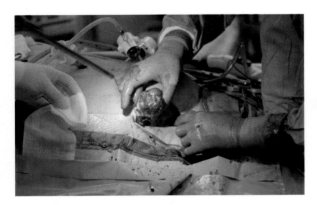

FIG. 12

Specimen removal

Right Kidney

The right colon is dissected from Gerota's fascia, and the duodenum is mobilized (Kocher maneuver). Then, the left hand is passed under the inferior, lateral, and superior kidney side to free the specimen while the LigaSure 5 mm (set at III 01/01) aids with the dissection (Fig. 10).

> **TIP**
>
> *The instrument is introduced through the umbilical port.*

The ureter is clipped and transected.

When approaching the pedicle, the optic is placed in the supraumbilical port, and the suction device is placed in the left lateral port (Fig. 10). The renal vascular pedicle is carefully dissected, clipped, and transected.

Left Kidney

The monitor is placed at the left side of the patient, the assistant moves to the right, and the instruments table is placed behind the surgeon. The left colon is dissected from Gerota's fascia. Then, the left hand is passed under the inferior, lateral, and superior kidney side to free the specimen while the LigaSure 5 mm (set at III 01/01) aids with the dissection.

> **TIP**
>
> *Care must be taken to avoid spleen damage while releasing the left kidney.*

The ureter is clipped and transected. The renal vascular pedicle is carefully dissected, clipped, and transected.

Bilateral Ureterectomy

When performing an associated bilateral ureterectomy, the surgeon moves to the patient's left side while the assistant is repositioned to the right. The laparoscopic cart is positioned at the patient's feet. A 5-mm trocar is inserted four fingerbreadths to the right of the umbilicus and approximately in line with the contralateral third port. The optic is placed in the supraumbilical port, the bipolar grasper is placed at the left-side port,

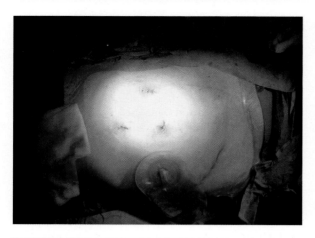

FIG. 13
Final result

Postoperative Considerations

The nasogastric tube is removed at the end of the procedure, and the intravenous perfusion is stopped on day 1. Pain is usually controlled with scheduled intravenous analgesics, which are replaced by the oral route after 24 hours. A light diet can generally be resumed on day 1 after surgery. The Foley catheter is removed on day 1 after surgery and the Penrose drain on day 2 after surgery. Patients leave the hospital on the third or fourth postoperative day and can resume normal light activities. Vigorous activities and heavy lifting are limited for at least one month after surgery.

Suggested Readings

1. Lipke MC, Bargman V: Limitations of laparoscopy for bilateral nephrectomy for autosomal dominant polycystic kidney disease. J Urol 2007 Feb; 177(2):627–631.

2. Ghasemian SR, Pedraza R: Bilateral laparoscopic radical nephrectomy for renal tumors in patients with acquired cystic kidney disease. J Laparoendosc Adv Surg Tech A 2005 Dec; 15(6):606–610.

3. Luke PPW, Spodeka J: Hand-assisted laparoscopic resection of the massive autosomal dominant polycystic kidney disease. Urology 2004 Feb; 63(2):369–372.

4. Lee DI, Clayman RV: Hand-assisted laparoscopic nephrectomy in autosomal dominant polycystic kidney disease. J Endourol 2004 May; 18(4):379–382.

5. Gill IS, Kaouk JH: Laparoscopic bilateral synchronous nephrectomy for autosomal dominant polycystic kidney disease: the initial experience. J Urol 2001 Apr; 165(4):1093–1098.

the monopolar scissors are placed at the umbilical port, and the suction device is placed at the right-side port (Fig. 11).

Kidney Extraction

The kidneys are removed through the lower ilioinguinal incision, and the laparoscopic bag is not needed (Fig. 12).

Closure of the Abdominal Wall

The abdominal wall is closed using running Vicryl 2-0 SH 1 Plus (needle ½ 21.8 mm) for the peritoneum, Vicryl 0 suture in "X" for the muscle, and a running Vicryl 1 CT Plus (needle ½ 39.9 mm) for the aponeurosis. Once the abdominal wall is closed, pneumoperitoneum is re-established, and the optic is introduced for revision of the hemostasis. A silicone Penrose drain is inserted. After evacuation of the pneumoperitoneum and removal of the trocars, the aponeurosis of the 11-mm port is closed with a Dexon II HGU-46 suture. The skin incisions are closed with subcuticular Monocryl 3-0 C 423 (Fig. 13).

Chapter 12

Laparoscopic Promontory Fixation

Contents

Introduction

Genitourinary prolapse occurs when the mechanisms for vaginal and uterine support begin to wear off. The most common prolapse is cystourethrocele, followed by uterine descent and rectocele. The correction of symptomatic moderate and severe genitourinary prolapse by the laparoscopic promontory fixation technique consists of placing two polyester (PET) meshes that pull the prolapsed bladder and rectum up. The distal part of the anterior mesh is fixed at the anterior vaginal wall, and the posterior mesh is fixed distally at the levator ani muscle bilaterally. The proximal part of the anterior and posterior mesh is anchored to the sacral promontory. The posterior dissection extends deep into the rectovaginal space, and the transperitoneal laparoscopic access allows for a good visualization of the operative field, as opposed to the open procedure.

Preoperative Preparation

The patient is admitted to the hospital the day before the surgery for bowel preparation, which includes 2 L of Colopeg® (1 envelope/L) p.o. and a Fleet® enema. Fasting starts at midnight before surgery. Thromboprophylaxis is implemented with good hydration, placement of compressive elastic stockings on the lower extremities, and low-molecular-weight heparin. Enoxaparin (Clexane®, Lovenox®) 40 mg sc 1 × day or nadroparin (Flaxiparine®, Fraxiparin®) 0.6 mL sc 1 × day is initiated on day 1 after the surgery and continued daily until the patient is discharged from the hospital. In selected cases, the treatment is continued for 30 days after the procedure. Patients also receive antibiotic prophylaxis with a single preoperative dose of intravenous second-genera-

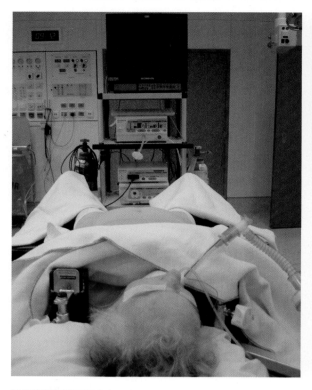

FIG. 1
Shoulder support

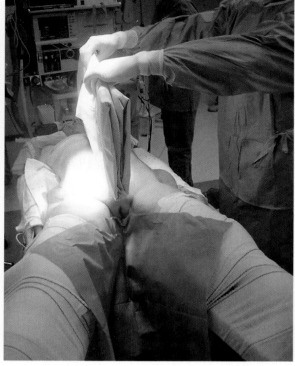

FIG. 2
Placement of the drapes

tion cephalosporin, unless they are allergic to penicillin. Blood type and crossmatch are determined.

Patient Positioning and Initial Preparation

The surgery is performed under general anesthesia. The patient is placed in the supine position with the lower limbs in abduction, allowing the laparoscopic cart to be moved toward the surgeon and intraoperative access to the perineum. The lower buttocks must be placed at the distal end of the operating table. The upper limbs are positioned alongside the body to avoid the risk of stretch injuries to the brachial plexus and to allow for free movements of the operative team. Shoulder support over the acromium clavicular joint is placed for the Trendelenburg position (Fig. 1).

A nasogastric tube is placed by the anesthesiologist and the stomach decompressed to allow additional space for the placement of the small bowel above the promontory. An 18Fr Foley catheter with 10 mL in the balloon is introduced after placement of the sterile drapes (Fig. 2).

The surgeon and the second assistant operate from the patient's left side, and the first assistant is placed at the opposite side of the surgeon. The laparoscopic cart is positioned at the patient's feet, while the instruments table and the coagulation unit are positioned at the left side of the patient.

Trocars and Laparoscopic Instruments

- 2×11 mm (optic 0° and bipolar grasper)
- 2×5 mm (scissors and suction device)

- Monopolar round-tipped scissors, bipolar grasper, dissector, 5-mm suction device, needle drivers (2), and 10-mm laparoscopic optic 0°

- Polyester multifilament mesh (Fig. 3)

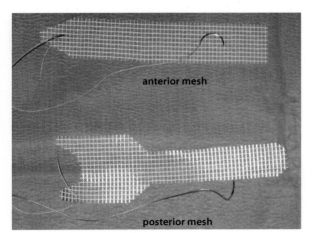

FIG. 3
Polyester mesh

Access and Port Placement

See Figure 4.

Veress Needle

A cutaneous incision is made at the inferior margin of the umbilicus, and the Veress needle is introduced through the incision (see Chap. 1, Veress Needle Introduction).

TIP

The incision should be 50% larger than the diameter of the trocar.

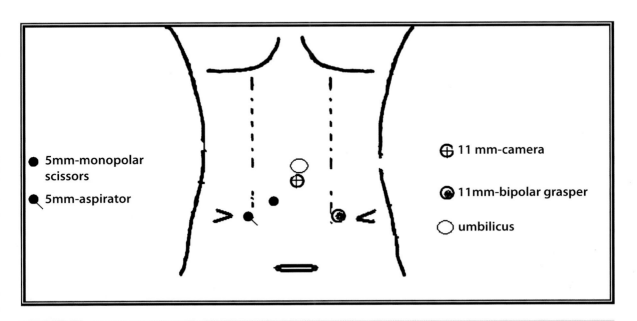

FIG. 4
Access and port placement (This figure was published in Wein: Campbell-Walsh Urology, 9th ed., Copyright Elsevier)

The insufflation tubing is connected to the Veress needle, the stopcock is opened, and insufflation is initiated.

> **TIP**
>
> *It is recommended to start with low flow to avoid damage to a vital structure in case the needle is malpositioned. Switch to high flow if the pressure of insufflation is increasing at a steady and normal level and there is also a tympanic percussion of the liver area.*

First Port (11 mm, optic 0°)

Once pneumoperitoneum is established, the needle is removed, and the 11-mm trocar is introduced through the same incision, perpendicularly to the abdominal wall.

> **TIP**
>
> *Pneumoperitoneum is established with an intra-abdominal pressure higher than 10 mmHg.*

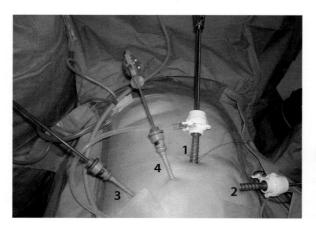

FIG. 5
Camera (1); Bipolar grasper (2); Suction device (3); and Scissors (4)

The optic is inserted through the trocar, and the insufflation line connected to it.

Second Port (11 mm, bipolar grasper)

A cutaneous incision is made 2 cm medial to the left anterior superior iliac spine for introduction of the 11-mm trocar.

> **TIP**
>
> *During trocar introduction, once the cutting tip pierces the peritoneum, it secures the position of the device, allowing further gliding of the trocar to a desired site. This maneuver prevents blockage of the movements of the working instruments following an incorrect insertion.*

Third Port (5 mm, suction device)

A cutaneous incision is made 2 cm medial to the right anterior superior iliac spine for introduction of the 5-mm trocar.

Fourth Port (5 mm, monopolar round-tipped scissors)

For insertion of the 5-mm trocar, a cutaneous incision is made at a point situated at the junction of the lateral 2/3 and medial 1/3 distance between the right anterior superior iliac spine trocar and the umbilicus trocar (see Fig.5).

> **TIP**
>
> *Pay attention to the epigastric vessels, which can be visualized by pressing the right lateral part of the abdomen.*

The operating table is moved down and backward, and the patient is placed in an extended Trendelenburg po-

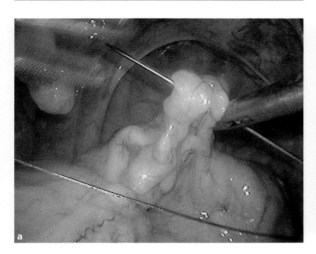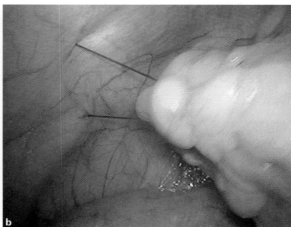

FIG. 6

a Suture through appendices epiploicae. **b** External fixation of the sigmoid to abdominal wall

sition. Steps are placed under the surgeon, and the bipolar and monopolar pedals are placed over the step. The surgeon, positioned higher than the assistant, can then use the working instruments (bipolar grasper and monopolar scissors) without being restrained by the assistant holding the optic in the upper midline position. This maneuver reduces the conflict between the operative team's arms.

Surgical Technique

Bowel Displacement

The sigmoid is positioned above the promontory by gently pushing back the loops of small bowel with the aid of the Trendelenburg position. If necessary, the cecum is dissected off the posterior peritoneum to increase its mobility and facilitate cranial displacement of the small bowel.

TIP

When facing difficulties retracting the bowels or when the patient cannot handle the extended Trendelenburg position, a fifth trocar (5 mm) can be introduced in the right iliac fossa, and a bowel retractor can then be used by the second assistant.

The sigmoid and its mesocolon are laterally displaced and fixed to the abdominal wall using a monofilament suture of 2-0 straight needle (Fig. 6a,b).

TIP

The suture needle is introduced through the skin at a point lateral and caudal to the left port, placed through the appendices epiploicae of the sigmoid colon, and exited close to the entrance point to be tied externally.

A valve is introduced into the vagina to aid in the exposure of the Douglas cul-de-sac and to facilitate the dissection of the rectovaginal and vesicovaginal plane (Figs. 7 and 8).

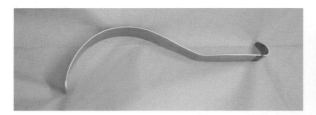

FIG. 7
Vaginal valve

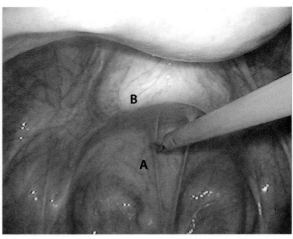

FIG. 8
Douglas cul-de-sac (A); Valve in the vagina (B)

Subtotal Hysterectomy and Anexectomy

If a subtotal hysterectomy with anexectomy is performed, the ureters are identified coursing down into the pelvis. The ovary is grasped and tractioned upward to better expose the infundibulopelvic ligament. The pedicle is then fully coagulated with the aid of the bipolar grasper and cut with monopolar scissors (Figs. 9a,b and 10a,b).

The dissection continues to expose the round ligament, which is coagulated and cut (Fig. 11).

The anterior and posterior leaves of broad ligament are dissected down to the vesicouterine fold and cut close to the uterus. The vesicoperitoneal fold is lifted and incised, mobilizing the bladder off the vagina. The uterine vessels are visualized and cut following coagulation with the bipolar grasper (Fig. 12).

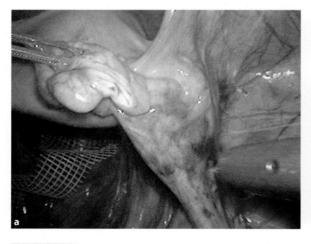

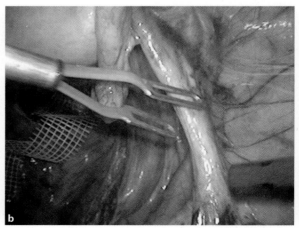

FIG. 9
a Infundibulopelvic ligament. **b** Bipolar coagulation

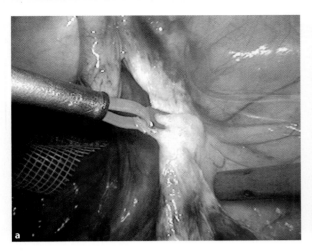
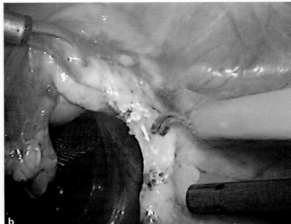

FIG. 10

a Infundibulopelvic ligament coagulated. **b** Ligament transected

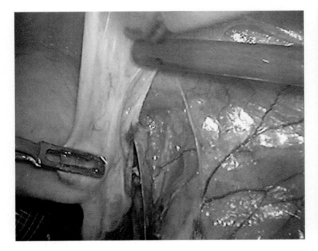

FIG. 11
Round ligament

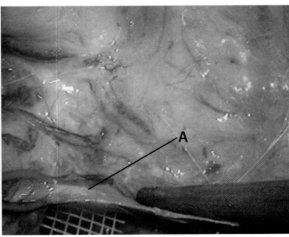

FIG. 12
Uterine artery (A)

TIP

In case of bleeding, applying traction to the tissue reduces the blood flow, and bleeding then can be controlled with the bipolar grasper.

The same procedure is done at the other side, and the uterus is transected with monopolar scissors above the cervix (Fig. 13).

The specimen is then placed higher than the level of the promontory to be removed at the end of the procedure.

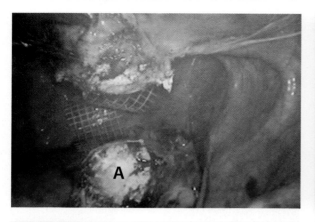

FIG. 13
Transected cervix (A)

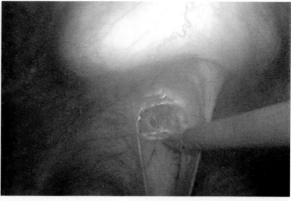

FIG. 14
Douglas pouch incised

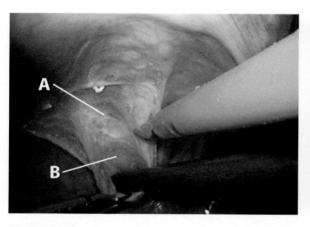

FIG. 15
Correct plane of dissection (A); Wrong plane of dissection (B)

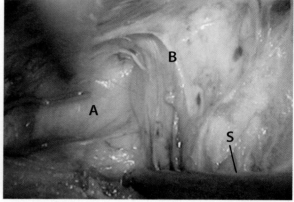

FIG. 16
Levator ani muscle (A); Rectum (B); Suction device (S) at the inferior part of the dissection

Posterior Dissection (Rectovaginal Plane)

When the uterus is in place, it must be mobilized off the pelvic cavity for the posterior dissection. The uterus is then fixed to the anterior abdominal wall using a monofilament 2-0 straight needle suture that transfixes its body.

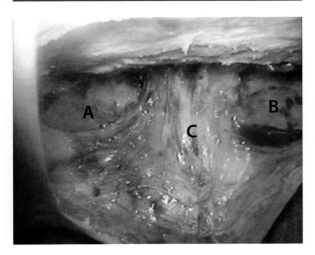

FIG. 17

Left (A) and right (B) levator ani muscles; Rectum (C)

> **TIP**
>
> *The suture needle is introduced through the skin at a midline point above the pubis, placed through the uterus, and exited close to the entrance point to be tied externally.*

The valve is inserted inside the vagina and is lifted to expose the Douglas pouch. The posterior peritoneum is grasped by the bipolar grasper and is placed under traction. The peritoneum is incised close to its superior deflection, and the inferior peritoneal lip with the fatty tissue attached is pulled down to expose the correct plane of dissection (Fig. 14).

> **TIP**
>
> *Two planes of dissection are encountered at this level. The right one is between the fatty tissue and the vagina, and by applying downward traction, the avascular plane of loose areolar tissue is exposed (Fig. 15). The wrong plane of dissection is between the fatty tissue and the rectum, and by following this plane, the chance of rectum injuries increases.*

The vagina is dissected from the rectum up to the level of the canal anal. The superior plane is followed laterally to arrive at the lateral wall of rectum, exposing the levator ani muscles bilaterally (Figs. 16 and 17).

> **TIP**
>
> *The assistant positions the suction device at the inferior part of the dissection and pushes down on the tissue at every step of the dissection to facilitate access to the right plane.*

Fixation of the Posterior Mesh

Following exposure of the levator ani muscle, the posterior mesh is introduced through the left 11-mm trocar, and it is bilaterally fixed to the uppermost part of the muscle using Ti-Cron® 2-0 sutures (needle ½ 26 cm).

> **TIP**
>
> *The position of the needle on the needle holder is 2/3 posterior and at a 45° angle. To insert the needle on the muscle, it first must be pushed in to load the needle onto the tissue. Then, the needle is turned, and the other needle holder is positioned below the exit point of the needle, grasping and fixing its tip (Fig. 18a,b). Finally, the needle is removed from the muscle following its curvature to prevent rectum damage.*

> **TIP**
>
> *The knot must be loosely tied to avoid postoperatory pain at the level of the anus.*

The broad part of the prosthesis is spread out over the rectum and placed as close to the vaginal deflection as possible (Fig. 19).

The Douglas pouch's peritoneum is closed using a U-shaped running suture of Vicryl 0. The mesh

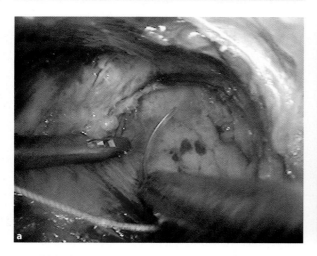
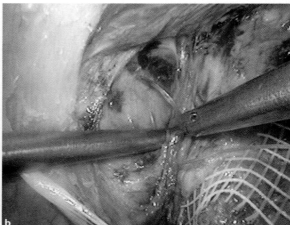

FIG. 18

a Needle position for the right side. **b** Needle position for the left side

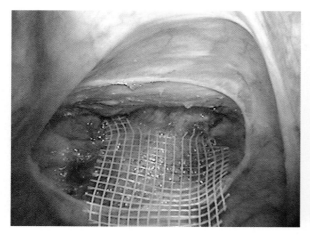

FIG. 19

Posterior mesh over rectum

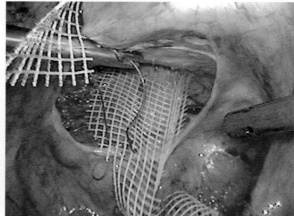

FIG. 20

Closure of posterior peritoneum

is included in the suture, fixing it to the peritoneum (Fig. 20).

Anterior Dissection (Vesicovaginal Plane)

The valve is introduced into the vagina and is lifted to put traction on the peritoneum. The peritoneum of the vesicouterine fold is transversely incised to expose the avascular plane of loose areolar tissue that separates the posterior surface of the bladder and the anterior vaginal wall (Fig. 21).

> **TIP**
>
> *The muscle fibers of the anterior vagina wall must be preserved to decrease the risk of mesh erosion.*

The dissection of this plane is carried out along the midline and extends laterally and inferiorly to the bladder trigone, taking care not to injure the bladder, vagina, or ureter.

> **TIP**
>
> *The ureter courses anteromedially after it passes under the uterine vessels, progressing toward the trigone of the bladder through a fascial tunnel on the anterior vaginal wall. In case the bladder or the vagina is accidentally opened, a running Vicryl 0 suture is used for repair.*

Fixation of the Vaginal Mesh

The anterior mesh is introduced through the left 11-mm trocar. After the mesh is spread out to cover the anterior vaginal wall, it is fixed to the apex and bilateral anterior vaginal wall using running Ti-Cron 2-0 sutures (needle ½ 26 mm) (Fig. 22a,b).

> **TIP**
>
> *The suture should not transfix the vaginal wall.*

If a subtotal hysterectomy is performed, the uterine cervix is also incorporated in this suture.

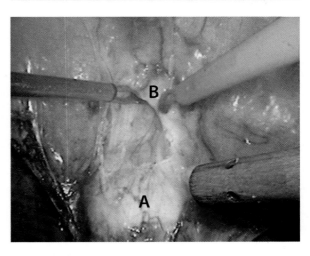

FIG. 21
Valve in the vagina (A); Bladder (B)

> **TIP**
>
> *When the uterus is left in situ, the mesh is partially divided. Each arm of the anterior mesh is passed through the broad ligament at the level of the isthmus on both sides of the organ, but from a safe distance from the uterine vessels. In case of asymmetric prolapse, the cervix can be slightly displaced to compensate for the asymmetry. In this case, the suture is placed at different levels on both sides of the cervix.*

Exposure of the Promontory

The promontory is either visualized or felt by palpation with the tip of the instruments. A longitudinal incision is performed on the posterior prevertebral parietal peritoneum to expose the anterior vertebral or presacral ligament, taking particular care not to injure the iliac vessels and the presacral (medium sacral vein) vessels. The incision on the peritoneum is then extended from the promontory to the right side of the Douglas pouch

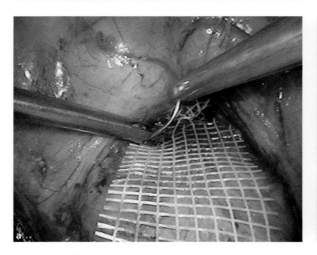

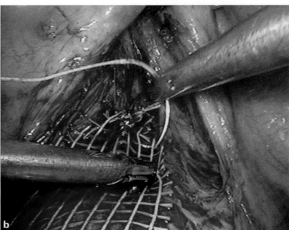

FIG. 22

a Left-side fixation. **b** Right-side fixation

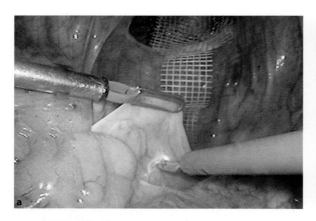

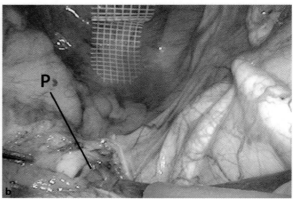

FIG. 23

a Promontory dissection. **b** Promontory (P) exposed

to further cover the mesh at the end of the procedure (Fig. 23a,b).

TIP

The "true horizon" of the optic must be correctly placed at this time to avoid unintentional dissection of the right common iliac artery instead of the promontory.

Promontory Fixation

A full-length Ti-Cron 1 suture (needle ½ 37 mm) is passed through the presacral ligament.

TIP

The position of the needle on the needle holder is 1/3 anterior and at a 45° angle.

The needle must be inserted from the right to the left with small and continuous movements of the needle on the anterior vertebral ligament (Fig. 24).

> ### TIP
>
> *The needle is introduced from right to left and with small movements because the left common iliac artery is more laterally located at this site, and the point of exit of the needle is less controlled than the entrance point.*

The needle runs only through the fibrous layer of the aponeurosis, avoiding perforation of the disc itself and the risk of iatrogenic spondylodiscitis.

After passing the suture, traction is applied to the thread to check that it is solidly anchored. The needle is positioned facing the head of the table and passed first through the posterior mesh and then passed through the anterior mesh. The needle charged with both prosthesis and with the tip facing the optic is placed at the promontory, simulating a hook, to determine the tension at the anterior and posterior mesh (Fig. 25a,b).

The right needle holder secures the meshes at the promontory while the left needle holder tests the tension. The posterior mesh *should have no tension*, and it should follow the curvature of the sacrum to respect the physiological movement of the Douglas pouch, avoiding postoperatory dyschesia. The anterior mesh should have medium tension applied to it, and the exact tension is confirmed by touching the mesh with the left needle holder. The knot is done extracorporeally using a half-hitch type knot (Weston knot). By passing both

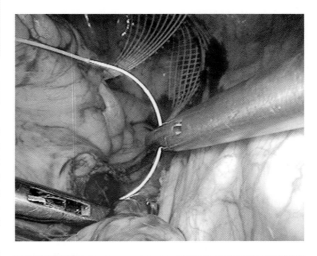

FIG. 24
Needle position for promontory fixation

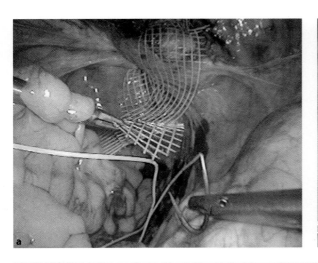

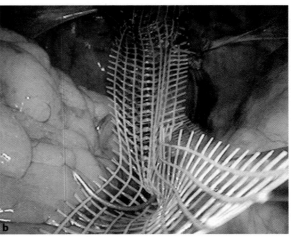

FIG. 25
a Needle position. **b** Mesh held in place

ends of the suture line through the right paraumbilical port (5 mm), the loose knot is descended through the port to the promontory. Then, the left needle holder grasps and pulls down the knot, and with the aid of the right needle holder, the knot is tied in place at the level of the promontory. Another four intracorporeal knots fix the mesh in place.

Closure of the Posterior Peritoneum

The posterior peritoneum and the peritoneum of the vesicouterine cul-de-sac are closed with a running suture of Vicryl 0. If the uterus is left in situ, the peritoneum covering the bladder is initially closed followed by the posterior part. In hysterectomized patients, a single running suture is done.

> **TIP**
>
> *The order of the posterior peritoneal suture is the following: (1) right distal edge of peritoneum, (2) right side of the mesh, (3) right side of the peritoneum covering the bladder, (4) left side of the peritoneum covering the bladder, (5) left side of the mesh, and (6) left distal edge of posterior peritoneum.*

The first knot is done, and then a running cranially oriented suture is performed, taking care to pass the needle at the edge of the peritoneum to avoid transfixing the ureter at the level of the promontory. The goal is to leave the mesh in a subperitoneal position to avoid small-bowel complications (Fig. 26a,b).

The aponeurosis of the 11-mm port is closed with a Polysorb 0 suture, and the skin is closed with running intradermic Monocryl 3-0.

Postoperative Considerations

The nasogastric tube is removed at the end of the procedure. The patient is given appropriate analgesia as per protocol (intravenous paracetamol during the first 24 h and major analgesics administered if necessary). The intravenous perfusion is stopped on day 1 after surgery, and a light diet can generally be resumed on the same day. The bladder catheter is removed on the second postoperative day. An osmotic laxative is prescribed for a few months and normal activity is resumed four weeks after the surgery.

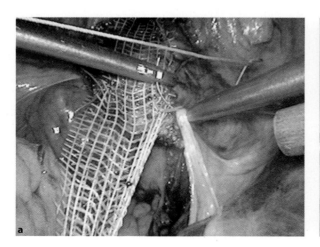
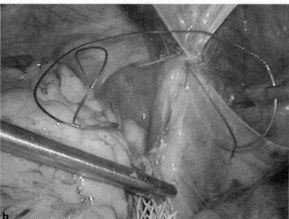

FIG. 26

a Posterior peritoneal closure. **b** Mesh covered by peritoneum

Schematic mesh position

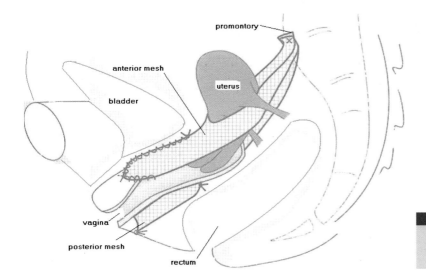

promontory

anterior mesh

uterus

bladder

vagina

posterior mesh

rectum

FIG. 27

Schematic mesh position (By permission of T. Darnies, Sofradim Production)

Suggested Readings

1. Rozet F, Mandron E: Laparoscopic sacral colpopexy approach for genito-urinary prolapse: experience with 363 cases. Eur Urol 2005 Feb; 47(2):230–236.

2. Grynberg M, Dedecker F: Laparoscopic sacral colpopexy: comparison of nonresorbable prosthetic tape (Mersuture) and a SIS collagen matrix (Surgisis ES). Prog Urol 2005 Sep; 15(4):751–755; discussion 755.

3. Antiphon P, Elard S: Laparoscopic promontory sacral colpopexy: is the posterior, recto-vaginal, mesh mandatory? Eur Urol 2004 May; 45(5):655–661.

4. Bruyere F, Rozenberg H: Laparoscopic sacral colpopexy: an attractive approach for prolapse repair. Prog Urol 2001 Dec; 11(6):1320–1326 [Article in French].

5. Paraiso MF, Falcone T: Laparoscopic surgery for enterocele, vaginal apex prolapse and rectocele. Int Urogynecol J Pelvic Floor Dysfunct 1999; 10(4):223–229.

Chapter 13

Extraperitoneal Laparoscopic Prostatic Adenomectomy

Contents

Introduction

Extraperitoneal laparoscopic prostatic adenomectomy is a straightforward surgery indicated for the treatment of symptomatic benign prostatic hyperplasia (BPH) in patients with large-volume glands. The access and initial operative steps are the same as for extraperitoneal laparoscopic radical prostatectomy (see Chap. 5). Minimal bleeding and hence reduced transfusion rate, shorter hospitalization, and faster recovery are additional advantages. This minimally invasive technique is a reasonable and effective alternative to open prostatectomy.

Preoperative Preparation

Before a patient consents to a laparoscopic prostatic adenomectomy, it is important to discuss the specific risks of the surgery, including the potential need to convert to the traditional open operation if difficulties arise.

The patient is admitted to the hospital the day before the surgery for bowel preparation, which includes 2 L of Colopeg® (1 envelope/L) p.o. and a Fleet® enema. Fasting starts at midnight before surgery. Thromboprophylaxis is implemented with good hydration, placement of compressive elastic stockings on the lower extremities, and low-molecular-weight heparin. Enoxaparin (Clexane®, Lovenox®) 40 mg sc 1 × day or nadroparin (Flaxiparine®, Fraxiparin®) 0.6 mL sc 1 × day is initiated on day 1 after the surgery and continued daily until the patient is discharged from the hospital. In selected cases, the treatment is continued for 30 days after the procedure. Patients also receive antibiotic prophylaxis with a single preoperative dose of intravenous second-generation cephalosporin, unless they are allergic to penicillin. Blood type and crossmatch are determined.

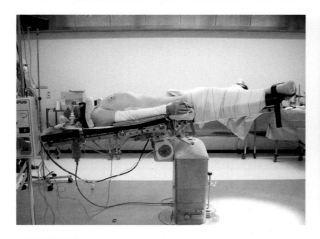

FIG. 1
Patient position

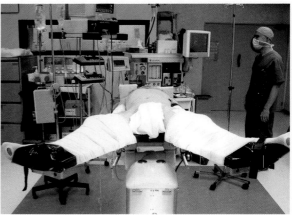

FIG. 2
Position of the legs

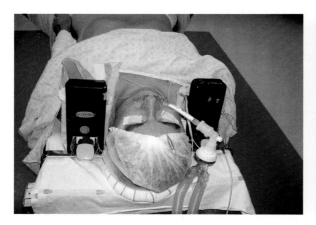

FIG. 3
Shoulder support

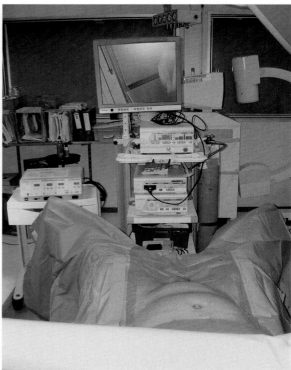

FIG. 4
Laparoscopic cart at patient's feet

Patient Positioning and Initial Preparation

The surgery is performed under general anesthesia. The base of the table must be positioned below the patient's hip to avoid elevation of the abdomen while in the Trendelenburg position (Fig. 1).

The patient is placed in the supine position with the lower limbs in abduction, allowing the laparoscopic cart to be moved closer to the surgeon and intraoperative access to the perineum (Fig. 2).

The lower buttocks must be placed at the distal end of the operating table. The upper limbs are positioned alongside the body to avoid the risk of stretch injuries to the brachial plexus and to allow for free movements of the operative team. Shoulder support is properly positioned for the Trendelenburg position (Fig. 3).

A nasogastric catheter is placed by the anesthesiologist and the stomach decompressed to allow additional space during extraperitoneal insufflation. The abdomen, pelvis, and genitalia are skin prepared in case conversion to an open procedure is required. An 18Fr Foley catheter with 10 mL in the balloon is introduced after the placement of the sterile drapes.

The surgeon and the second assistant operate from the patient's left side, and the first assistant is placed at the opposite side of the surgeon. The laparoscopic cart is placed at the patient's feet, while the instruments table and the coagulation unit are positioned at the left side of the patient (Fig. 4).

Trocars and Laparoscopic Instruments

- 2 × 11 mm (optic 0° and bipolar grasper)
- 3 × 5 mm (scissors, suction device, and palpator)
- Monopolar round-tipped scissors, bipolar grasper, dissector, 5-mm suction device, needle drivers (2), and 10-mm laparoscopic optic 0°

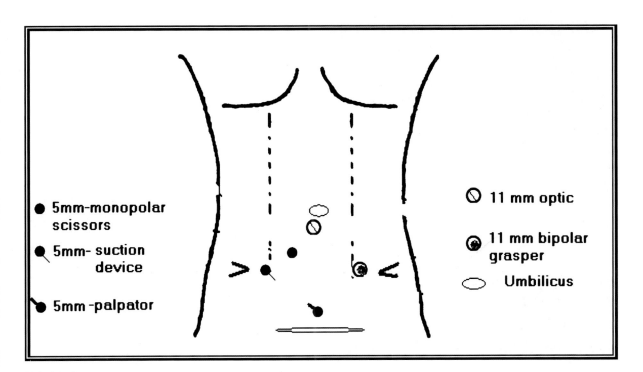

FIG. 5

Access and port placement (This figure was published in Wein: Campbell-Walsh Urology, 9th ed., Copyright Elsevier)

Access and Port Placement

The access and port placement is the same as for extraperitoneal laparoscopic radical prostatectomy – see Chapter 5, Figure 5.

Final Position of Trocars

The operating table is moved down and backward, and the patient is placed in a slight Trendelenburg position. Steps are placed for the surgeon, and the bipolar and monopolar pedals are placed over the step (Fig. 7a,b).

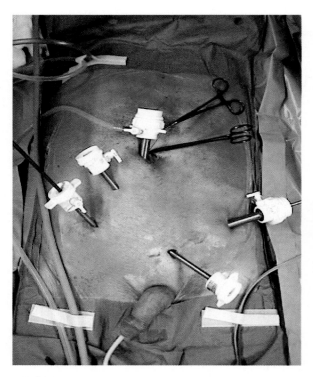

Surgical Technique

Peritoneum Displacement and Exposure of the Bladder Neck

The peritoneum is cranially mobilized to increase the extraperitoneal space. The fibroareolar and fatty tissue layers between the superolateral aspect of the bladder and the medial aspect of the external iliac vein are bilaterally released. This maneuver, along with reduction of any visible pelvic wall hernia, allows for further peritoneum displacement.

> **TIP**
>
> *Every effort should be made to thoroughly coagulate the bleeding vessels during this dissection to avoid image decay throughout the procedure.*

The fatty tissue around the prostate is freed, starting laterally from the reflection of the endopelvic wall toward the midline on both sides (Fig. 8).

The fibroareolar and fatty tissue attached at the level of the Santorini plexus and over the anterior surface of the prostate are pulled down toward the bladder neck with gentle but firm traction with the bipolar grasper. The superficial branch of the deep dorsal vein complex is coagulated with the bipolar grasper and cut with the cold scissors (Fig. 9).

> **TIP**
>
> *The superficial branch is transected at a safe distance from the pubic bone to prevent retraction of the vein and to permit easy vessel control in case of bleeding.*

The maneuver of downward traction and pulling of the fatty tissue continues until resistance is encountered, signaling the approach of the bladder neck. The dissected fatty tissue is then lifted and divided in the midline to facilitate the coagulation and transection of the vessels that overlie the bladder neck. The fatty tis-

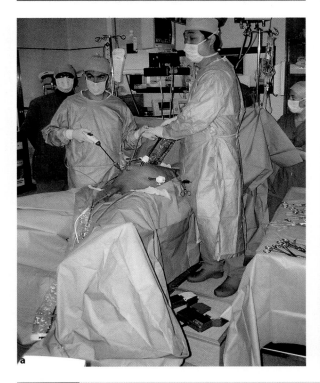

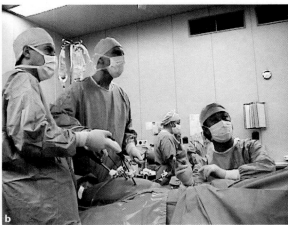

FIG. 7

a Steps under the surgeon. b Operative team's position

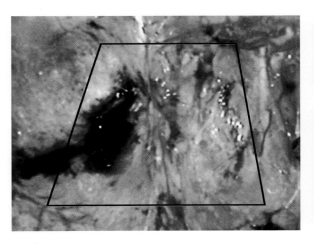

FIG. 8

Fatty tissue around the prostate

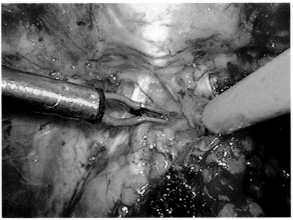

FIG. 9

Coagulation of the superficial branch of the deep dorsal vein complex

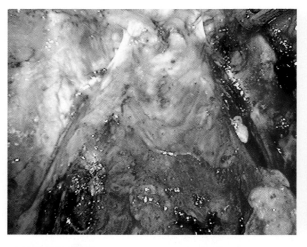

FIG. 10
Anterior prostatic surface free of fatty tissue

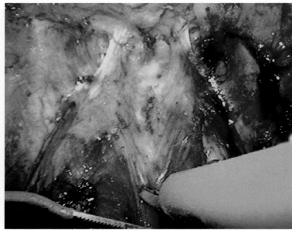

FIG. 11
The bladder neck is situated under the crossing of the fibers of the puboprostatic ligaments

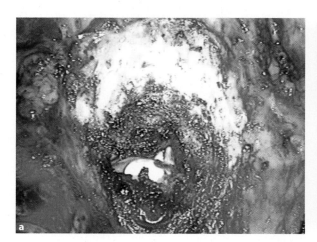

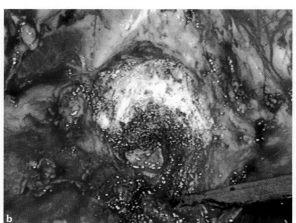

FIG. 12
a Bladder neck opened with catheter inside. **b** Catheter removed

sue removal facilitates visualization and dissection of the bladder neck (Fig. 10), which is usually located under the crossing of the fibers of the puboprostatic ligaments (Fig. 11).

Bladder Neck Dissection and Division

A transversal incision with the monopolar scissors along with forceful counter pressure with the bipolar grasper, which is placed over the bladder, opens the su-

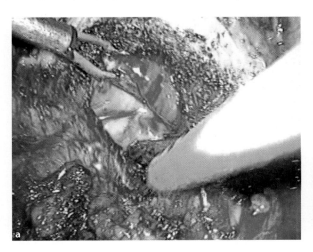

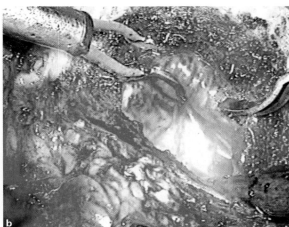

FIG. 13

a Medium lobe. **b** Plane of dissection – medium lobe

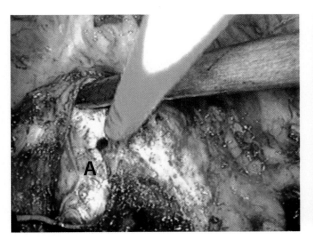

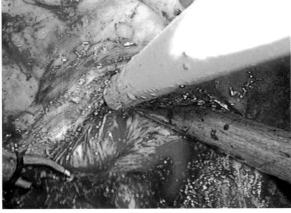

FIG. 14

Adenoma (A) – lateral lobe enucleation

FIG. 15

Anterior dissection of lateral lobes

perficial layer and exposes the correct plane of dissection. The anterior aspect of the urethra is exposed and incised. The catheter is removed, and the locations of the ureteral orifices, bladder neck, and adenoma are determined (Fig. 12a,b).

Adenoma Dissection

A transverse incision is made at the mucosa of the bladder neck, and the monopolar scissors are used to dissect

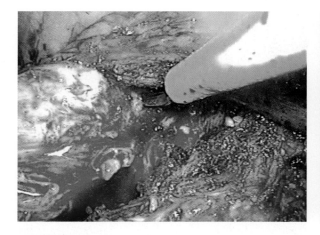

FIG. 16

Right lateral lobe is released

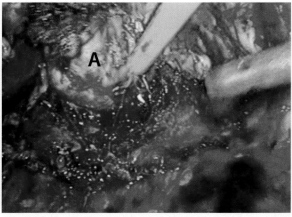

FIG. 17

Adenoma (A) is rolled to the side

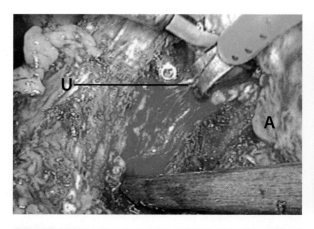

FIG. 18

Urethral mucosa (U) incised and adenoma (A) removed

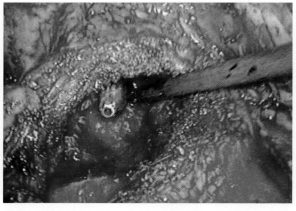

FIG. 19

Empty prostatic fossa

the median lobe (if present) from the overlying prostatic capsule (Fig. 13a,b).

The dissection is deepened posteriorly to the level of the adenoma and extended sideways to permit complete enucleation of the lateral lobes (Fig. 14).

Once a well-defined plane is developed, the grasper instrument lifts the prostatic capsule to further develop the plane. The anterior commissure at the apex is in-

cised, separating the lateral lobes of the prostate anteriorly (Fig. 15).

The urethral mucosa over the right lateral lobe is incised at the level of the apex, and the right lateral lobe is released (Fig. 16).

The left lateral lobe is freed by the same approach, and care should be taken not to injure the muscle fibers of the external urinary sphincter.

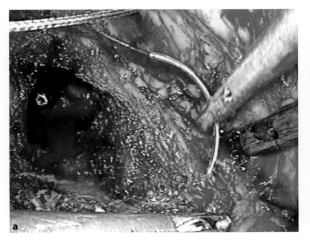

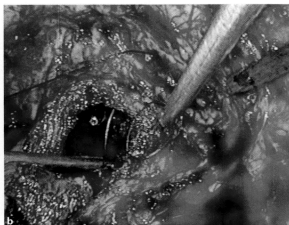

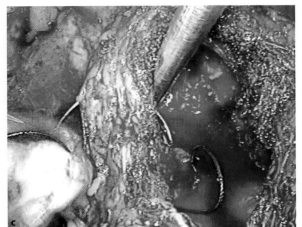

FIG. 20

a Right lateral capsular suture. **b** Needle exiting inside prostatic fossa. **c** Left lateral capsular suture

It is important to grasp the adenoma, rolling it to the sides to facilitate the dissection (Fig. 17).

Posteriorly, the dissection is advanced proximal to the verumontanum; the urethral mucosa is incised, and the adenoma is removed (Fig. 18).

Prostatic Fossa Hemostasis

The prostatic fossa is inspected to confirm that the adenoma has been completely removed (Fig. 19).

A full thickness interrupted suture of Vicryl 0 is placed at the lateral sides of the prostatic capsule (at the 9 and 3 o'clock positions) to secure hemostasis (Fig. 20a–c).

The bladder mucosa is then advanced into the prostatic fossa and sutured at the 6 o'clock position with

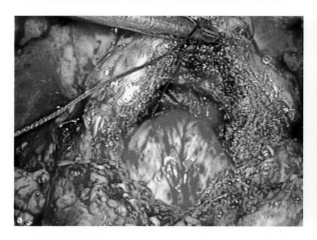
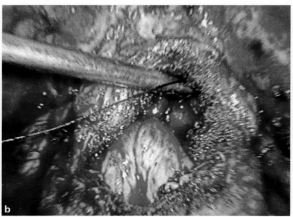

FIG. 21

a Bladder mucosa advanced into prostatic fossa. **b** Trigonization of prostatic fossa

Vicryl SH 2-0, followed by bilateral full thickness interrupted sutures that complete the trigonization of the prostatic fossa (Fig. 21a,b).

> **TIP**
>
> *Pay attention to the ureteral orifices when performing these sutures.*

Closure of the Prostatic Capsule

A 22Fr three-way Foley catheter with a 30-mL balloon is inserted through the anterior urethra and prostatic fossa into the bladder (Fig. 22).

The balloon is initially filled with 10 mL. Starting at the left side, the prostatic capsule is closed with full thickness running sutures of Polysorb 2-0 GL 123 (needle ½ 26 mm) (Fig. 23a,b).

> **TIP**
>
> *A long suture thread should be used.*

The balloon is now filled with 30 mL and positioned inside the bladder. Continuous irrigation with saline solution is initiated to avoid blood clot formation.

An EndoCatch® bag is introduced through the left 11-mm port, and the adenoma is placed into the bag. The prostate is removed by enlarging the left iliac spine port site.

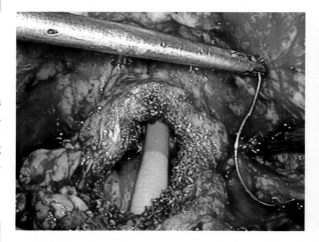

FIG. 22

Foley catheter inside bladder

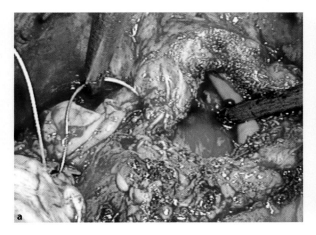
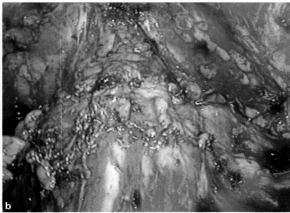

FIG. 23
a Closure of the prostatic capsule. **b** Final result

A Penrose drain is placed close to the prostate capsule and exited through the right iliac spine port site. The aponeurosis of the 11-mm ports is closed with Polysorb 0 UL 877 sutures (needle 5/8), and the skin is closed with a running intradermic Monocryl 3-0. The Penrose is sutured to the skin with Flexidene 2-0, and the skin incisions are covered with Opsite® bandages. The urethral catheter is secured to the leg.

Postoperative Considerations

The patient is given appropriate analgesia as per protocol, including intravenous paracetamol during the first 24 h and major analgesics administered as necessary. The intravenous perfusion is stopped on day 1, oral fluids are started the morning after surgery, and a light diet can generally be resumed on day 1. The drain is usually removed after 48–72 h or after secretions are below 50 mL. The irrigation of the bladder is suspended on postoperative day 1 or 2 and the bladder catheter is removed on day 3 if urine is clear. When residual haematuria persists, a cystogram is performed. Normal activity is resumed four weeks after surgery.

Suggested Readings

1. Baumert H, Ballaro A: Laparoscopic versus open simple prostatectomy: a comparative study. J Urol 2006 May; 175(5):1691–1694.
2. Porpiglia F, Terrone C: Transcapsular adenomectomy (Millin): a comparative study, extraperitoneal laparoscopy versus open surgery. Eur Urol 2006 Jan; 49(1):120–126.
3. Rehman J, Khan SA: Extraperitoneal laparoscopic prostatectomy (adenomectomy) for obstructing benign prostatic hyperplasia: transvesical and transcapsular (Millin) techniques. J Endourol 2005 May; 19(4):491–496.
4. Van Velthoven R, Peltier A: Laparoscopic extraperitoneal adenomectomy (Millin): pilot study on feasibility. Eur Urol 2004 Jan; 45(1):103–109.

Subject Index